Pregnancy Cookbook for First Time Dads

A pocket guide to answer to first time moms cravings

By

Eve C. Bird

Copyright

Disclaimer

The information in this book is only meant to be used for general reading. Even though every effort has been made to make sure the information is correct, the author and publisher do not promise or guarantee that it is full, correct, reliable, useful, or available. If you use this kind of information, you do so at your own risk.

The author and distributor are not responsible for any harm, loss, or damage that may come from using this book. For certain scenarios, it is best to get help from a professional.

Any group, service, or product mentioned in this book is only meant to be informative and does not mean that the author endorses or recommends it. Some things in this book might be changed at any time.

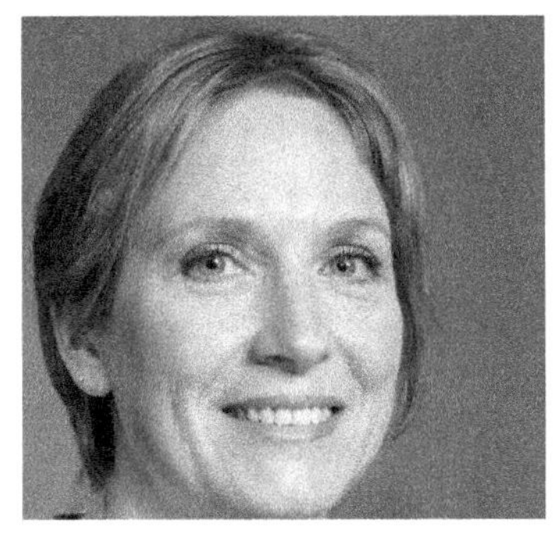

About the Author

Eve C. Bird is a well-known authority in the fields of skincare, dietetics, exercise, and health. She is passionate about enabling people to live healthy, balanced lifestyles. She has become a reliable voice in the quest for holistic well-being because of her vast expertise gained from in-depth research and real-world experience. Her devotion to disseminating practical knowledge has positively impacted many lives and established a community of people committed to adopting a better, healthier way of living. Readers learn the transformative power of conscious decisions and uncover the keys to glowing health and wellness with the help of Eve C. Bird.

INTRODUCTION

Food and pregnancy

The experience of becoming pregnant is amazing and full of many emotions and changes. As a new life develops inside the mother's womb, it's an exciting and wondrous period. It seems as though a miraculous process begins at conception and lasts for nine months, growing from a single cell to a little human being.

Pregnancy is a remarkable physical experience. The body undergoes numerous modifications in order to support the developing kid. In order to accommodate the growing baby, the uterus enlarges, hormone levels rise, and blood volume rises. However, these adjustments also bring about a variety of aches and pains, exhaustion, and morning sickness, which can occasionally make things difficult.

However, pregnancy involves more than simply physical changes; it's an emotional rollercoaster. There's a lot of happiness and excitement, but there are also anxious and uncertain moments. The first time you feel those first kicks and hear the baby's heartbeat, these experiences will leave you feeling incredibly connected and in love.

It's critical to have the support of family members and medical professionals throughout this time. Check-ups during pregnancy, guidance on diet and exercise, and simply having a confidante to chat to can all be really beneficial. It all comes down to having constant support and attention.

Pregnancy is ultimately a journey of love and growth. It's about developing as a person and a parent, not simply a baby. And in the end, all of the difficulties are worthwhile because of the happiness that comes with welcoming a new life into the world.

Food plays a crucial role during pregnancy, not only for the health of the mother but also for the development and well-being of the growing baby. Eating a balanced and nutritious diet is essential to support the increased nutritional needs of both mother and fetus during this important time.

First and foremost, adequate nutrition during pregnancy is vital for the baby's growth and development. The nutrients obtained from food serve as the building blocks for the baby's organs, tissues, and overall growth. Key nutrients such as folic acid, iron, calcium, protein, and essential vitamins contribute to the healthy development of the baby's brain, bones, and vital organs.

Folic acid, for example, plays a critical role in the early stages of pregnancy in preventing neural tube defects such as spina bifida. Iron is essential for the production of red blood cells, which transport oxygen to both the mother and the baby. Calcium is necessary for the development of the baby's bones and teeth, while protein supports overall growth and development.

In addition to supporting the baby's growth, a well-balanced diet during pregnancy also helps to maintain the mother's health and well-being.

Pregnancy places increased demands on the mother's body, and proper nutrition can help prevent complications such as anemia, gestational diabetes, and pre-eclampsia. Adequate intake of nutrients also supports the mother's energy levels, immune function, and overall vitality during this physically demanding time.

Furthermore, good nutrition during pregnancy can have long-lasting effects on the health of both the mother and the child. Research has shown that a mother's diet during pregnancy can influence the baby's future health outcomes, including their risk of chronic diseases such as obesity, diabetes, and cardiovascular disease later in life. By prioritizing healthy eating habits during pregnancy, mothers can lay the foundation for their child's lifelong health and well-being.

It's important to note that every pregnancy is unique, and nutritional needs may vary depending on factors such as age, weight, medical history, and lifestyle. Consulting with a healthcare provider or a registered dietitian can help expectant mothers develop a personalized nutrition plan tailored to their specific needs and preferences.

Food during pregnancy is about so much more than just calories and nutrients. It's about nurturing your baby, supporting your own health, and savoring this incredible journey into motherhood. So, eat well, listen to your cravings (within reason!), and remember that every bite you take is a step towards a healthy, happy pregnancy for you and your little one.

CHAPTER 1: The Basics of Nutrition for Mom and Baby

Pregnancy causes a number of physical and hormonal changes to your body, as you undoubtedly already know. You'll need to choose healthy foods from a range of sources to nourish both you and your developing child.

Consuming a nutritious, well-balanced diet will make you feel good and supply all the nutrients you and your child require. Since your diet is your baby's primary source of nutrition, it's imperative that you consume all the nutrients that your body requires.

The positive aspect? These nutritional recommendations offer a variety of delectable options and are all quite easy to follow. You can quickly put together a nutritious menu, even in the face of cravings (hot sauce on peanut butter, anyone?).

An increase in nutrients

It should come as no surprise that while you are pregnant, your body requires more nutrients because you are growing a whole new person! The saying "eating for two" isn't totally true, although you do need additional macro- and micronutrients to sustain both you and your child.

- **Micronutrients**: are dietary elements like vitamins and minerals that are needed in comparatively small quantities.

- **Macronutrients**: Calorie-dense or energy-producing nutrients. We are discussing fats, proteins, and carbs. During pregnancy, you'll need to consume more of each kind of nutrient.

Based on your needs, the following general recommendations on a few crucial nutrients will need to be modified:

Nutrient	Daily requirements for pregnant women
calcium	**1200 milligrams (mg)**

folate	600–800 micrograms (mcg)
iron	27 mg
protein	70 and 100 grams (g) daily, up each trimester

Most expectant mothers can choose a diet that includes a range of healthful foods, such as the following, to suit their increased nutritional needs:

- complex carbohydrates and protein
- fats that are good for you, such as omega-3s, vitamins, and minerals

How much and what to eat

Consume a diverse range of foods to meet both your needs and those of your infant. It's just a little more intense than a typical healthy eating regimen. Actually, you should carry on eating regularly throughout the first semester, then as your baby grows, increase your daily caloric intake by 350 in the second trimester and 450 in the third.

Steer clear of highly processed junk food as much as possible. For example, soda and chips have no nutritional benefit. Fresh produce, fruits, and lean meats like chicken, fish, beans, or lentils are better for you and your child. This does not imply that you should abstain from all of your favorite foods when you are expecting. Simply counterbalance them with wholesome foods to ensure you don't overlook any vital vitamins or minerals.

Protein

A baby's tissues and organs, including the brain, depend on protein to grow properly. Additionally, it promotes the formation of uterine and breast tissue during pregnancy. It even contributes to your blood supply growing, which makes it possible for your kid to receive more blood.

Every trimester of pregnancy increases your demand for protein. Studies indicate that pregnant women should consume much more protein than is already advised. Time to start serving more jerk chicken, salmon teriyaki, and shrimp fajitas.

Depending on your weight and the stage of your pregnancy, you should consume between 70 and 100 g of protein each day. To find out how much you precisely need, speak with your doctor.

Among the best places to get protein are:

- lean pork and beef
- peanut butter
- chicken
- salmon
- almonds beans with cottage cheese

Calcium

Calcium controls how much fluids your body uses and aids in the development of your baby's bones. A pregnant woman should take 1,000 mg of calcium daily, preferably in two 500 mg doses. Regular prenatal pills won't be enough to complement your calcium needs.

Among the best places to get calcium are:

- low-mercury seafood
- dairy products
- canned light tuna
- shrimp
- catfish
- salmon dark green
- leafy vegetables that are calcium-set tofu

Folate

Also referred to as folic acid, folate is a vital component in lowering the risk of neural tube abnormalities. These are serious birth disorders, like spina bifida and anencephaly, that impact the baby's brain and spinal cord.

The American College of Obstetrics and Gynecology (ACOG) suggests consuming

600–800 micrograms of folate each day while you are pregnant. Folate is present in the following foods:

- liver
- nuts
- almonds
- peanut butter
- leafy veggies dried beans
- lentils eggs

Iron

Iron increases blood flow in conjunction with potassium, salt, and water. This makes it more likely that you and your child will receive enough oxygen.

It is recommended that you consume 27 mg of iron daily, ideally in combination with vitamin C to improve absorption. Suitable sources for this vitamin consist of:

- lush
- dark green vegetables
- breads or cereals enhanced with citrus fruits
- lean meat and eggs from chicken

Note:

During your pregnancy, you need additional nutrients such as choline, salt, and B vitamins to stay healthy.

In addition to eating healthfully, it's critical to take prenatal vitamins and drink at least eight glasses of water every day. Certain minerals, such as iron, choline, and folate, are hard to get enough of from diet alone.

Make sure you discuss the prenatal vitamins you should take with your physician.

Food Fix: Pregnant and What to Eat

Food aversions and cravings: You may develop food aversions during pregnancy, which means you won't enjoy the flavor or aroma of certain foods. Additionally, you might be desiring one or more food kinds.

Cravings during pregnancy: You may develop a strong need for doughnuts, Chinese food, or an unusual fusion of foods, such as ice cream and pickles.

The reason behind food aversions or desires in pregnant women is unknown. Nonetheless, scientists think hormones are involved.

It's acceptable to occasionally give in to these cravings, particularly if they are for items that are included in a balanced diet. Nonetheless, you ought to make an effort to consume fewer processed and junk food items.

Usually, there's a delicious substitute that's a better choice. Do you have a craving for fries? With so many beneficial elements, oven-roasted sweet potato wedges can feel just as decadent.

Aversions to certain meals may, however, only become troublesome during pregnancy if those foods are crucial to the growth and development of the unborn child.

If you have negative side effects from foods you should be eating during pregnancy, consult your doctor. To make up for the nutrients you're not getting enough of in your diet, your doctor may recommend additional meals or supplements.

Pica

This disorder is characterized by cravings for non-nutritional foods. Among other weird foods, pregnant women with pica may wish to consume clay, cigarette ashes, or starch.

A pregnant lady experiencing pica may be experiencing a vitamin or mineral deficiency. If you have cravings for or have consumed nonfood products, it's critical to let your doctor know. Consuming such foods might be harmful to both you and your child.

Gaining weight healthily during pregnancy

Avoid overstressing yourself if weight gain is a worry. It's common to gain a little weight while pregnant. The baby receives nutrients from the excess weight. Additionally, some of it is kept in storage for nursing the newborn.

During pregnancy, women typically gain 25 to 35 pounds (lbs.). It's common to gain more weight if you were underweight before becoming pregnant, or to gain less weight if you start off heavier.

The ideal weight for you to gain during your pregnancy can be discussed with your doctor. Although every person is unique, the table below offers some broad recommendations.

Suggested weight increase for a single-child pregnant woman

Initial weight	Body mass index	Recommended increase in weight
underweight	18.5	28 to 40 lbs.
average weight	18.5 to 24.9	25 to 35 lbs.

overweight	25 to 29.9	15 to 25 lbs
obese	30.0	11 to 20 lbs.

Note: The formula to get body mass index (BMI) is weight (in pounds) / height (in inches)2 x 703.

The number on the scale shouldn't cause you too much concern. Focus on consuming a range of nutrient-dense foods rather than your weight. Eating a healthy diet is crucial, and dieting to reduce weight or stop weight gain can be bad for both you and your unborn child.

Exercise that's healthful

Exercise can help you manage your health and reduce stress during pregnancy, in addition to eating a diet that is focused on nutrition.

Walking and swimming are also excellent ways to begin active. Select a hobby (or hobbies!) that you love.

Steer clear of contact sports and extreme sports like basketball and rock climbing. The ideal situation is to go on while remaining safe.

If you were never an athlete before becoming pregnant, take it gently and don't push yourself too hard. For additional assistance, think about checking out some workouts or programs designed especially for expectant mothers.

In order to prevent dehydration, it's also critical to consume lots of water. Always let your physician guide you in your exercise regimen.

To ensure the best possible health for both you and your developing child, make sure you're eating a nutritious, well-balanced diet during your pregnancy. Eat more complete, nutrient-dense foods and less processed and quick food, which are low in nutritional content.

Consume these:

- healthy carbohydrates and protein at every meal and snack
- five servings or more of fruits and vegetables each day, dairy products, or foods high in calcium
- foods high in vital fats
- pregnancy supplements

Steer clear of these:

- alcohol

- high mercury fish, raw meats and shellfish, processed meats that aren't cooked, and excessive caffeine
- dairy products without additives

With the help of your healthcare team, develop a meal plan that is targeted, pleasant, and doable depending on your weight, age, medical history, and risk factors. This is something you can handle.

CHAPTER 2: Stocking the Dad-Friendly Pantry

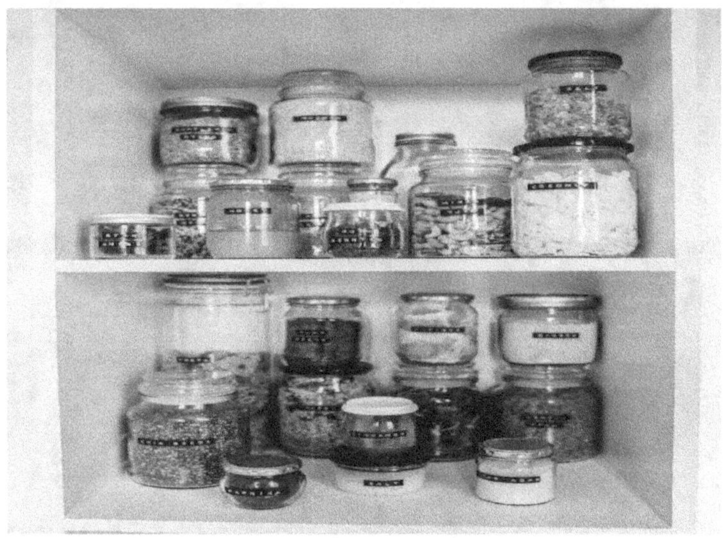

For many soon-to-be fathers, learning that their partner is expecting may be a very stressful moment. During the early stages of pregnancy, emotions might run wild and you might consider making changes to your diet, lifestyle, or even your living spaces.

For many women, the beginning of a pregnancy is also the ideal moment to consider what foods you have in your kitchen and how to use them to support healthy eating, prevent pregnancy symptoms, and manage any cravings that may arise.

Eating healthily when pregnant

First and foremost, it's critical to enlist the assistance and support of family members in this endeavor. Having someone who can relate to you and support you in making healthy changes can be really beneficial. We also like to eat the items that are easiest to get our hands on, so if your cabinets are stocked high with chocolates, crisps, and other sweets, you can bet that you'll be chowing down on them for the duration of your pregnancy!

1. Increase your supply of basics: Grains that you should stock your cupboards with in abundance include brown rice, buckwheat, quinoa, couscous, and wholewheat pasta. In addition to being high in energy, these foods also contain fiber and wholegrains, which help maintain the healthiest possible digestive system. They also contain protein, which is necessary for the development and maintenance of all bodily tissues, including the developing tissues of your growing child. These kinds of essentials also take little time to prepare, store in your cabinet for a long time, and are reasonably inexpensive to purchase. It's crucial, in my opinion, to eat some wholegrains with each meal every day.

Bread, chapattis, pitta breads, bagels, and English muffins are all excellent options to keep on hand. What's even better is that you can freeze these foods to extend their shelf life. Aim to always select whole grain versions of these foods to increase your intake of fiber, which is particularly crucial during the months of pregnancy.

2. Increase your nut intake: One of my favorite foods is nuts. In addition, they include a wealth of plant-based chemicals, vitamins, minerals, fiber, protein, and healthy fats! This tree nut nutrition comparison chart is always so helpful to me when I need to remind myself of how nutritious nuts are. You may learn more about the advantages of nuts for your health by visiting my blog.

In my opinion, nuts are the ideal prenatal snack, especially when combined with fruits. This is because fruits include vitamin C, which can actually enhance the absorption of any iron that may be present in the nuts. Nuts are the ideal food to help you stay fueled in between meals because they are pretty full and high in energy. Furthermore, nuts can serve as a crucial meat substitute in a vegetarian or vegan diet if you are expecting.

Keep in mind that nuts can have a high calorie content, therefore moderation is key while consuming them. About a handful is a portion. To assist you be more in control of exactly how many you eat, it could be useful to purchase them in compact grab-and-go packs or even move them to some small tupperware containers at home and take them with you. To cut down on extra fat and salt, it's also advisable to choose plain nuts most of the time.

3. Obtain some simple meals to snack on, particularly if you're feeling queasy: If you're feeling sick, it's best to stock up on simple foods. This is due to the fact that their bland flavor and dry texture can aid in containing them when a variety of other foods start to act as triggers. It's best to experiment with different plain foods to see what you enjoy for a snack. Use these when you truly need an energy boost, and make sure to check the label to make sure they are a good choice. Excellent choices consist of:

- crackers made of whole grains
- Sticks of bread
- cakes made of rice

- simple popcorn
- whole grain bread

4. Make your selections for decaf tea: It's advised that you limit your caffeine intake while pregnant. However, if you enjoy coffee or tea a lot, this may be difficult for you. Fortunately, there are many decaf options accessible in supermarkets and high street shops in the UK.

Try keeping your pantry stocked with your favorite decaf tea in addition to choosing more unusual varieties like fruit, herbal, and naturally decaffeinated teas like rooibos. To avoid getting too tired of the same tea, I like to do this and then just switch between them. I've discovered that when I'm pregnant, I typically start the day with decaf tea, move on to one or two Rooibos during the day, then choose a fruit tea or anything like a lemon and ginger blend at night. Keep an eye out for my blog post on herbal teas during pregnancy, which I'll be posting soon.

5.Utilize your freezer to its fullest: Many individuals are hesitant to include frozen fruits and vegetables in their meals, but in actuality, they can be just as nutritious, often even more so because they are frozen at their prime than fresh produce! They are also a highly affordable and practical way to keep nutritious foods that you can easily add to any meal to help increase nutritional intakes, fiber content, and meet some of your daily five! I cannot stress how important it is to stock up on them.

Using frozen choices can be a fantastic approach to try eating a couple of pieces of vegetables with lunch and dinner each day. An additional quick and simple method to incorporate fruits into your regular diet is to use frozen fruits in crumbles or oatmeal, for example.

6. Invest in a large oat bag: Not only are oats a naturally wholegrain, but they are also a highly adaptable ingredient that is high in proteins, fiber, and energy. Therefore, early in your pregnancy, one of my suggestions for stocking your cupboard with essentials is to purchase a large bag of plain or rolled oats! Oats are a staple in my daily routine. I enjoy them in porridge, as a topping for other cereals, or even in my wildly famous overnight oats dish.

Oats can also be used to make low-sugar energy balls, flap jacks, and oat bars, all of which are excellent snack options for on-the-go vitamin and energy boosts. I also like to add oats to puddings, like frozen forest fruits with natural yogurt and a dash of oats or flapjack squares.

7. Organize your spice cabinet properly: When it comes to enhancing the flavor of food during pregnancy, herbs and spices can be a godsend. During the second trimester of pregnancy, your unborn child will begin to taste and swallow flavors and substances from your food. Therefore, it's a good idea to concentrate on eating a nutritious diet and maybe consider cutting back on your intake of sugar and salt.

This is where herbs and spices come into play, making them an excellent substitute for sugar and salt in meals and cuisines. I've always believed that spices and herbs are underappreciated and don't get used nearly enough to flavor cuisine. A recipe will frequently call for "a pinch of salt," but it's not always necessary especially if you're willing to try out some more unusual herbs and spices.

I've been enjoying experimenting in the kitchen with herbs and spices ever since I became pregnant. They have always been a staple of my meals, but since I'm pregnant, I've also been experimenting with more spicy dishes and pushing myself a bit because I've never been great with spicy cuisine. I like them more than ever right now, for whatever reason.

8. Pulses, beans, and lentils in cans: Pulses, beans, and lentils are probably among the healthiest foods on the lists of many dietitians. Once more, these are wonderful foods that don't receive enough recognition. But these foods are also high in fiber, low in calories, and packed with nutrients like calcium, iron, and protein.

In addition to nuts, these items are essential for vegetarians and vegans, and most of us could use more of them in our diets.

It's a fantastic idea to stock up on them throughout pregnancy, especially canned beans of various kinds and lentils, which you can add to pies, curries, and tomato sauces. Because it's so simple, I also love to use chickpeas to make my own falafels and/or hummus.

Pulses, beans, and lentils are very nutritious, low-cost, and long-lasting foods that you can keep in your pantry. Another fantastic staple and perfect pregnancy meal or snack is beans on toast, especially if you need a little extra energy in the first trimester.

9. Raw produce: This is a great choice if you're fortunate enough to be able to afford to have delivery boxes of fresh produce sent right to your house every week, and it's even better if you're expecting.

If not, now more than ever you'll need the minerals, fiber, and hydration that come with eating plenty of these foods, so stock up on fresh fruit and vegetables. There's a good reason behind the adage "eat five or more fruits and vegetables a day": they're extremely beneficial to our health. Furthermore, the fiber they provide can also assist to lessen some of the digestive issues you might be experiencing while pregnant.

If you live with a spouse or family, it's a good idea to ask them to bring in a large quantity of fresh fruits and veggies once a week or so, so you have them for the following week. It is best to choose what suits your particular lifestyle at home, but personally, I like to stock up on Sundays so that I know what I have to work with for the rest of the week.

In the meanwhile, you can always count on some good old frozen and tinned meals to tide you over. If all else fails, consider using reliable online shopping to have your fresh goods delivered each week.

10. Purchase some jars and storage boxes: I adore showcasing my goods in storage jars and boxes like the ones in the image below. It's not only for show, though; I also think these make it much simpler to see what's left AND what's in your cabinets, which can help you stay inspired when it comes to mealtimes and food. Eating healthily on the road is also made a lot easier with smaller storage bins that you can carry with you. See my blog post about healthy snacks to eat while pregnant for further ideas.

CHAPTER 3: Dad's Quick and Healthy Breakfasts

It's likely that you've heard how vital breakfast is, and it is. While your doctor may urge you to follow a certain diet, you don't have to, but eating a healthy, balanced diet is crucial to ensuring that you and your developing baby get the vitamins and minerals you require. A nutritious breakfast during pregnancy is part of that.

Here, we'll look at some delicious, simple, and healthful pregnancy breakfast ideas as well as the reasons why eating breakfast is crucial.

These mouthwatering and wholesome pregnancy breakfast recipes will provide you and your unborn child the nourishment you need to start the day off right.

A few of our recipes are quite easy, making them ideal for hectic days spent at work or on the road. Additionally, there are some decadent options that are perfect for preparing, enjoying, and relaxing on the weekends or on days when you have a little more time to yourself.

What is a good breakfast during pregnancy?
As long as your breakfast is high in fiber and low in sugar, salt, and fat, you're on track for a healthy start to the day. Healthy breakfast

ingredients include:

- Wholegrain cereals

- Semi-skimmed milk.

- Fresh, frozen, or canned (with juice) Fruit

  Eggs

Smoothie with banana and blueberries

Smoothies are a great breakfast alternative since they are flavorful, simple to make, and loaded with important vitamins and minerals. You have the option of using fresh fruit or stocking your freezer with your favorite frozen foods, which will keep for longer.

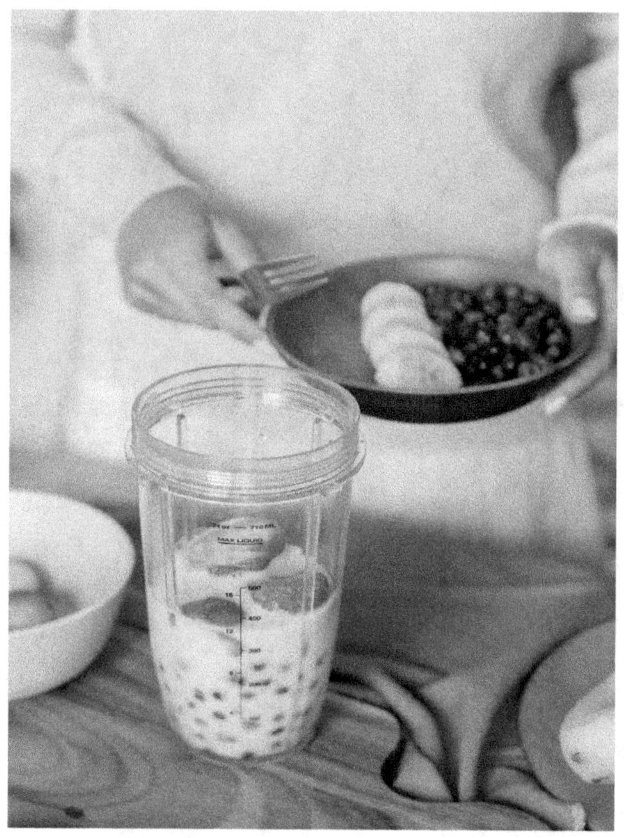

What you'll need is

- 150g of frozen or fresh blueberries

- One banana, peeled

- A generous portion of Greek yogurt (or a vegan substitute)

- One cup of apple juice

Technique

- Fill a blender with all of the ingredients.
- Blitz until desired level of smoothness is achieved.
- Transfer to a glass and savor!

You can save any leftovers in the refrigerator for a nutritious pregnancy snack.

Scrambled eggs

Scrambled eggs, a popular breakfast dish, are an excellent choice. This is due to the high protein content of eggs, as well as the presence of numerous vitamins and minerals. Remember that during your pregnancy, you should opt for British Lion hen eggs, which can be identified by the lion stamp, as well as hen eggs produced under the Laid in Britain scheme. This is because they are less likely to contain Salmonella.

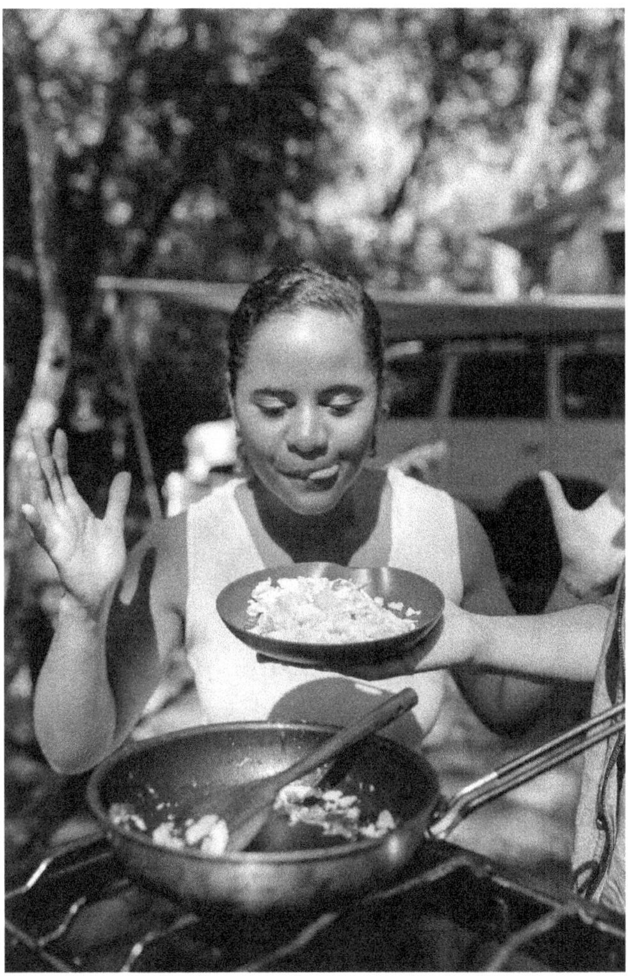

You'll need two eggs:

- 6–7 tablespoons of semi-skimmed milk.

- One knob of butter.

- A pinch of salt.

Method

- Get a bowl and mix the eggs and milk inside.
- Sprinkle a pinch of salt into the mixture.
- Melt the butter in a nonstick saucepan or frying pan, then add the egg mixture.
- Stir and fold until scrambled and well cooked throughout.
- Add more butter for a silkier texture.

To serve, pair with wholemeal bread and grilled tomatoes for a delicious breakfast.

Breakfast burrito

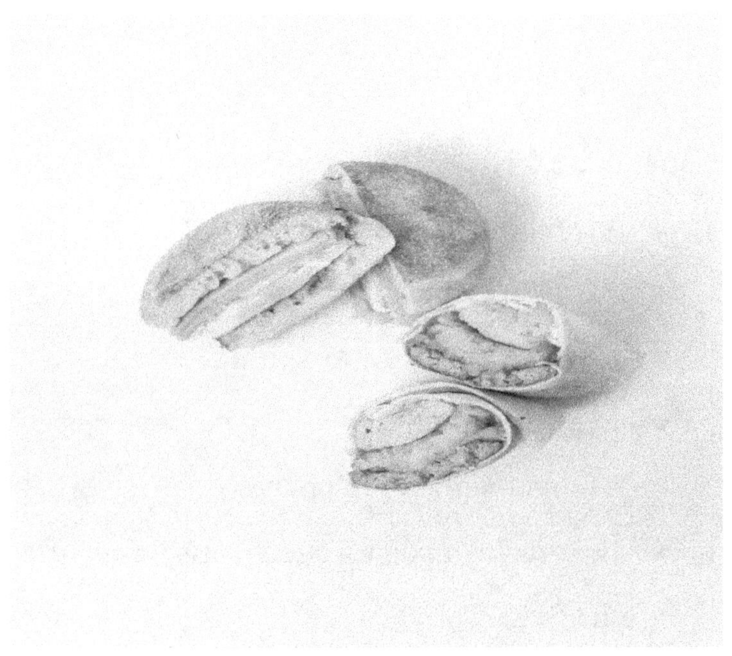

For a Mexican take on eggs for breakfast, consider a delightful pregnancy breakfast burrito. This delectable addition to your weekend breakfast routine has a variety of nutrients.

Here is a breakfast burrito recipe to get you started.

Serves 1

You'll need

- one wholemeal tortilla wrap.

- 2 eggs

- 1 tablespoon of semi-skimmed milk.

- 1 spring onion.

- 1 tomato and ¼ red pepper.

- 10 gram cheddar cheese (or dairy-free cheese).

- One dash of black pepper.

- One teaspoon of vegetable oil.

- A pinch of black pepper.

Method:

- Break the egg in a bowl, add milk and whisk together.

- Transfer the mixture to a nonstick frying pan heated with a teaspoon of oil.

- Fry gently until the mixture has set.

- Meanwhile, cut the spring onion, tomato, and red pepper and toss in a bowl with a pinch of black pepper.

- Once the egg is thoroughly cooked, remove from the pan and place on the tortilla.

- Top the egg with spring onion, tomato, pepper, and shredded cheese.

- Roll the tortilla into a burrito and lay it under a hot grill until the cheese melts.

Extra Tips

If you want something simpler, there are plenty of different pregnancy breakfast options to pick from.

Yogurt

Yogurt, whether natural, Greek, or dairy-free, is an excellent source of calcium and protein.

For a quick and healthy breakfast, simply top your favorite yogurt with fresh or tinned (in juice) fruit. You may even add a handful of granola for an extra crunchy treat, but make sure to check the sugar content.

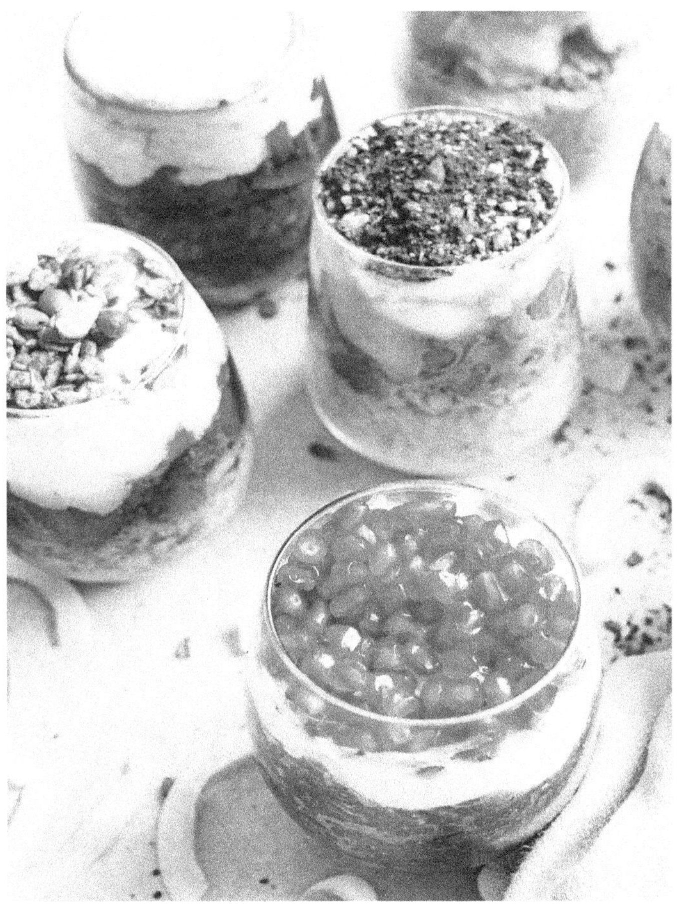

Cereals can be a healthy breakfast option during pregnancy, provided they are low in fat and sugar. Choose fiber-rich cereals like Bran Flakes, Weetabix, Shredded Wheat, and All Bran, and use semi-skimmed milk. A handful of fresh fruit might provide an additional nutritious boost.

Porridge with fruit

Sprinkle sliced bananas or berries over your cereal. If you don't have much time in the morning, consider making overnight oats the night before:

- Place the oats in a jar with milk, yogurt, and some sliced, frozen, or dried fruit.
- Refrigerate until the next morning.
- Vegan-friendly options include plant-based milk and yogurt.

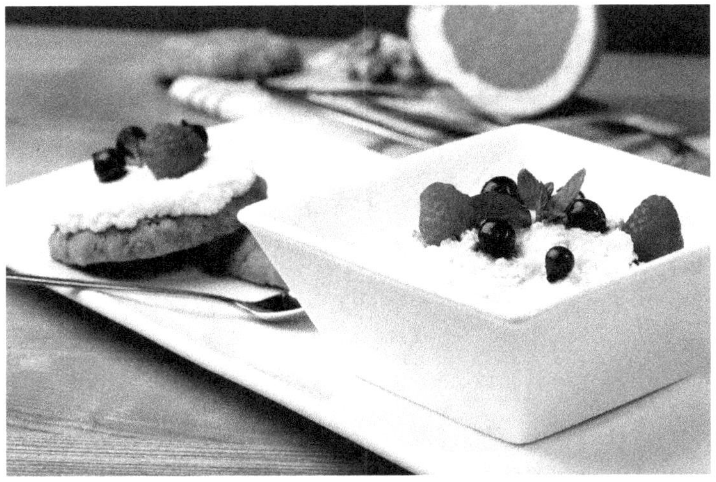

Be advised that a recommended serving size for oats is 30g, which is equivalent to 2 to 3 tablespoons (dry). This may not appear to be much, but when you add milk or water, it expands more than you would anticipate!

Avocado Toast

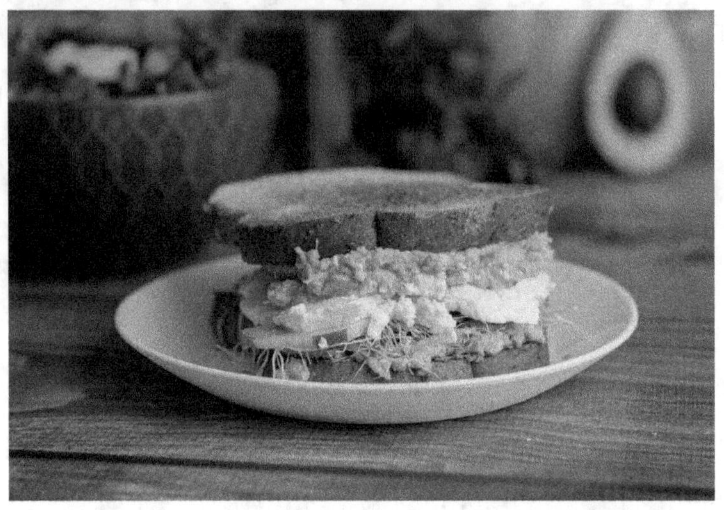

Avocado is one of the healthiest foods for pregnancy since it contains healthy fats, potassium, folate, vitamins B5, B6, C, E, and K. Slice avocados and mix them onto multigrain or whole wheat bread with chia or hemp seeds. You can also add cream cheese for added flavor and any other fruit for sweetness. This delightful breakfast is full of nutrients and flavor.

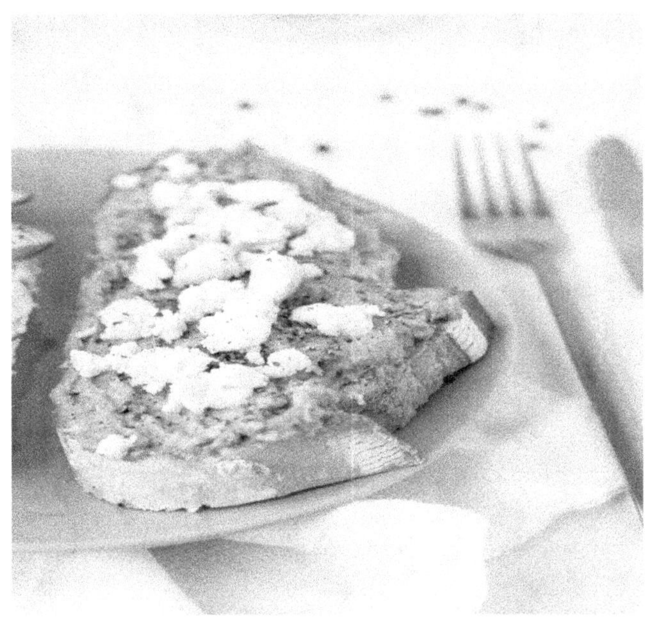

Ingredients:

- ½ small avocado.

- ½ teaspoon fresh lemon juice.

- ⅛ teaspoon kosher salt.

- ⅛ teaspoon fresh ground black pepper

- 1 slice of whole grain bread, toasted

- 1/2 teaspoon extra virgin olive oil

Garnish with Maldon sea salt or red pepper flakes (optional).

Directions:

- In a small bowl, combine the avocado, lemon juice, salt, and pepper
- Mash it with the back of a fork gradually.
- Top toasted bread with the avocado mixture.
- Drizzle with olive oil and add any desired toppings.

Quality ingredients are essential for making the ultimate avocado toast. Use fresh, crusty whole wheat bread and the finest extra-virgin olive oil you can find.

Nutritional Information (per serving):

- 200 Calories

- 13g fat, 18g carbs, 5g protein.

Ginger blueberry whole wheat pancakes

Ginger blueberry whole wheat pancakes: The entire family will like these.

Ingredients:

- Servings: 4
- 3/4 cup whole wheat flour.
- 1/2 tsp ground ginger
- 1/2 teaspoon ground cinnamon.
- 1 pinch of ground allspice.
- 1/2 teaspoon baking soda.
- 1/2 cup of apple juice concentrate.
- 1/4 cup milk.
- 1/2 tbsp butter melted
- 1 medium-sized egg

- 3/4 cup fresh blueberries.

- 1 teaspoon of canola oil.

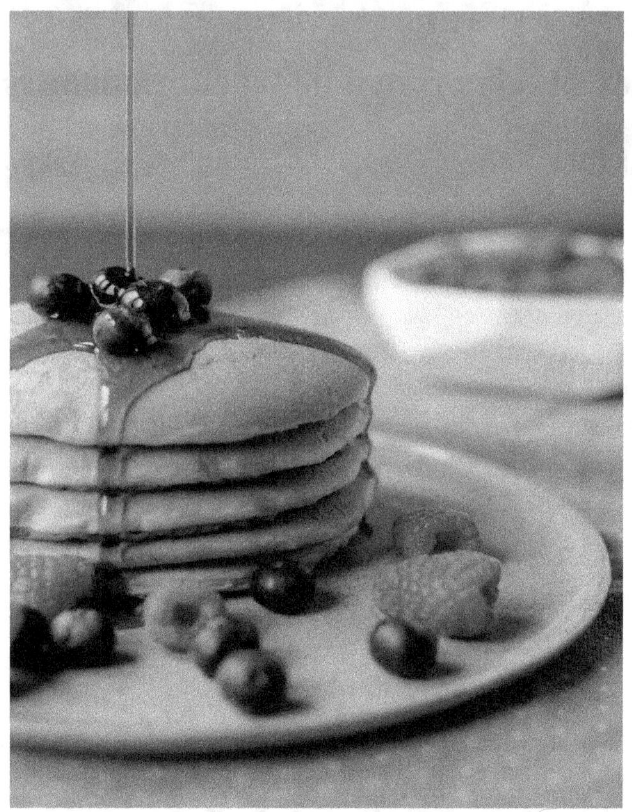

Method:

- Use a pancake mix, but make sure it's whole wheat and contains protein.

- Add flavor to the mixture by combining a teaspoon of ground ginger, a teaspoon of cinnamon, and a cup and a half of blueberries.

Blueberries are a nutrient-dense fruit high in antioxidants and vitamins, while ginger is a natural anti-nausea cure for morning sickness.

- Mix flour, ginger, cinnamon, allspice, and baking soda in a large mixing bowl. Set aside.

- In the second bowl, combine the juice, milk, butter, and eggs. Whisk to combine.

- Add the juice mixture to the flour mixture and whisk until combined.

- Add the blueberries and gently mix to incorporate.

- Heat 1/4 cup of canola oil in a skillet for each pancake.

- Cook 2-3 minutes till golden brown, then rotate and cook for 2 minutes.

Nutrition Facts: Per Serving: 100 g Amount: 1 serving

- Calories: 202.68 kcal (849 kJ).
- Calories from fat: 35.38 Kcal% Daily Value
- Total Fat: 3.93g, 6%.
- Cholesterol: 45.04mg15%
- sodium (187.86mg), 8%
- potassium (223.42mg).5%

- Total carbs: 37.28g12%

- sugars (15.09g) at 60%.

- Dietary fiber: 1.26g, 5%.

- Protein: 4.56g9%

- Vitamin C (29.1mg)49%

- Iron: 2.3mg

- Calcium: 13% (40.2mg) 4%

Ginger melon salad

Ginger melon salad is your go-to for B vitamins and vitamin C. Breakfast is as simple as slicing some fruit, and fruit salad is a delicious way to get your vitamins. Toss in a half-tablespoon of minced fresh ginger with your chopped melon (such as watermelon and cantaloupe, as well as grapes or any other fruits you want). To add even more flavor, mix with mint, juice concentrate, and lime zest. The key ingredient in this dish is really the fresh ginger – it adds a zing to the flavor. Use extra virgin olive oil and sea salt to enhance the taste as well.

Prep Time: 5 minutes
Cook Time: 0 minutes
Yield: 2 servings

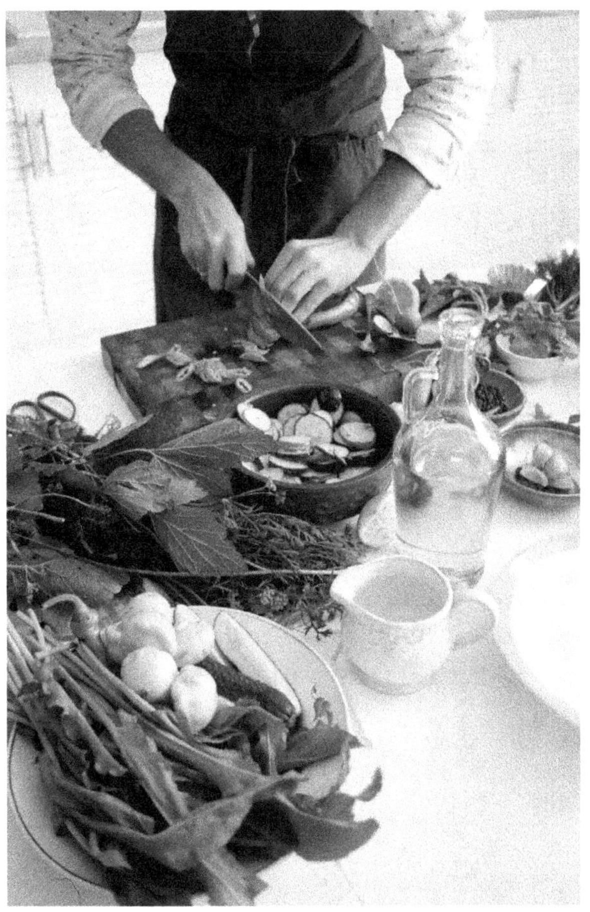

Ingredients:

2 large handfuls of salad leaves (or spinach)

1/2 small melon, cut into small chunks

1/2 small cucumber, peeled and cut into small chunks

1 Tablespoon fresh ginger, grated or diced into small pieces

2 teaspoons fresh lemon juice

2 Tablespoons extra virgin olive oil

1/2 teaspoon sea salt (or to taste)

Method

- Place the salad leaves in a bowl and add in the extra virgin olive oil.

- Sprinkle in the sea salt.

- Grate or dice some fresh ginger and add it into the salad.

- Squeeze in some fresh lemon juice to the melon salad.

- Dice the melon into small chunks and add to the bowl. I like to slice the melon and then cut it into small pieces.

- Dice some cucumbers into small pieces and add them into the bowl. The cucumber chunks should be cut to a similar size as the melon chunks. The cucumber adds extra crunch and makes the salad less sweet and more refreshing.

- Toss the salad really well – I like to just use my hands to get the ginger, sea salt, fresh lemon juice, and extra virgin olive oil really mixed in.

Nutrition:
- Calories: 172
- Sugar: 9 g

- Fat: 14 g
- Carbohydrates: 12 g
- Fiber: 3 g
- Protein: 3 g
- Cholesterol: 0 g

Carrot muffins

Carrot muffins are easy on the stomach and perfect for breakfast on the go. Healthy muffins are an excellent pregnancy breakfast option, and this carrot muffin recipe sounds delicious. Something about a homemade pastry, especially when it's still warm from the oven, just hits the spot. With ginger (our favorite morning sickness treatment), Greek yogurt for protein, and, of course, nutritious carrots, this meal will keep you going for hours and also makes an excellent afternoon snack.

To make these carrot muffins, you will need the following ingredients:

- Carrots, of course. They make the muffins extremely moist and lend a delicious, earthy carrot cake flavor. Shred them using the big holes of a box grater.

- All-purpose flour, whole wheat flour, and almond flour - Whole wheat flour provides the muffins a whole grain flavor, while all-purpose and almond flour keep them moist and tender.

- Baking powder and eggs make the muffins puff up while baking.

- Cinnamon, nutmeg, ginger, and vanilla provide a warm, spicy depth of taste.

- Almond milk - or whatever milk you choose! My own oat milk might also work great here.

- If you don't have avocado oil on hand, you can substitute another neutral oil in this recipe. Vegetable, grape seed, or canola oil all work well.

- Cane sugar makes the muffins slightly sweet.

- Walnuts For crunch

- Raisins provide a chewy texture and sweet flavor to these healthful carrot muffins.

- Whole rolled oats - I enjoy topping carrot cake with cream cheese frosting, but these carrot muffins? Not very much. Instead, I top them with oats for a nutritious finish. Also, use sea salt to bring out all of the tastes!

Ingredients measurement:

- 1 cup all-purpose flour, spooned and smoothed.
- ¾ cup whole wheat flour, measured and leveled.
- 1/2 cup almond flour, spooned and smoothed.
- 1 tablespoon of aluminum-free baking powder
- 1 teaspoon of cinnamon.
- ½ teaspoon ground ginger.

- ½ teaspoon nutmeg.

- ½ teaspoon sea salt.

- ⅔ cup unsweetened almond milk.

- 1/2 cup avocado or neutral oil.

- Two huge eggs.

- 1/2 cup cane sugar

- 1 teaspoon of vanilla extract.

- 3 cups shredded carrots

- 1/2 cup chopped walnuts.

- Add ½ cup raisins and ¼ cup whole rolled oats for topping.

Preparation Time: 15 minutes.

Cook Time: 20 minutes.

Total time is 35 minutes.

Serves twelve.

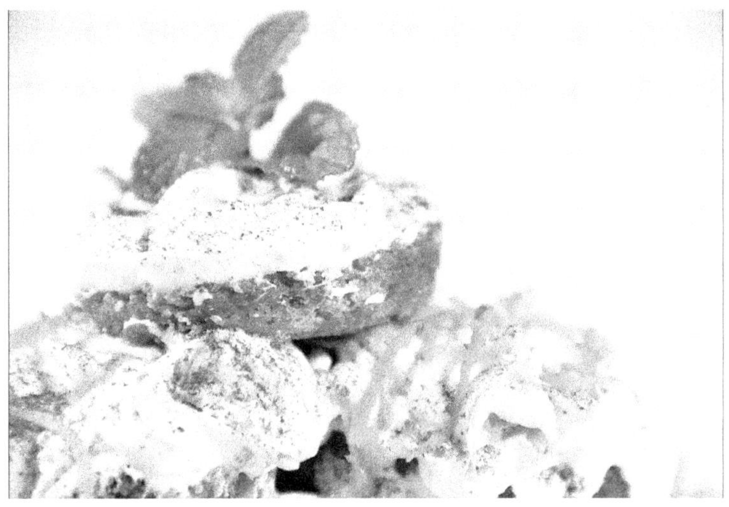

How To Make Carrot Muffins

This carrot muffin recipe is incredibly simple to make!

- Prepare the batter. In a smaller bowl, whisk together the dry ingredients.

- In a large basin, combine the wet ingredients.

- Mix the shredded carrots into the wet ingredients.

- Whisk the dry ingredients into the wet components until just incorporated.

- Be careful not to over-mix! If you do, the muffins will become dense. Fold in the walnuts and raisins.

- Next, divide the batter among the muffin cups. Use a 1/3-cup measuring cup to scoop the batter into a prepared muffin tray.

- Sprinkle the oatmeal on top of the muffins.

- And bake! Place the muffins in a 400°F oven and bake until the tops bounce back to the touch or a toothpick inserted into the center comes out clean.

- Allow them to cool in the pan for 10 minutes before transferring to a wire rack to finish cooling.

That is it! These carrot muffins are great for breakfast or a snack, or they can be served as part of a bigger brunch dish. They go well with savory breakfast dishes such as frittatas, breakfast casseroles, or scrambled eggs, as well as a large bowl of fresh fruit. If you have any leftover carrot muffins, keep them at room temperature for up to two days. After that, pop them in the freezer. They defrost well for a quick breakfast or nutritious snack!

Instructions:

- Preheat the oven to 400°F. Grease a 12-cup muffin pan.

- In a larger bowl, combine the flours, baking powder, cinnamon, ginger, nutmeg, and salt.

- In a large mixing bowl, combine the almond milk, oil, eggs, sugar, and vanilla. Stir in the carrots.

- Mix the dry ingredients into the wet ingredients, and mix together till it is properly combined. Fold in the walnuts and raisins.

- Using a ⅓-cup measuring cup, scoop the batter into muffin cups.

- Bake for 16–20 minutes, or until the muffin tops bounce back to the touch. Allow to cool for 10 minutes, then transfer to a wire rack to cool fully.

Granola bar

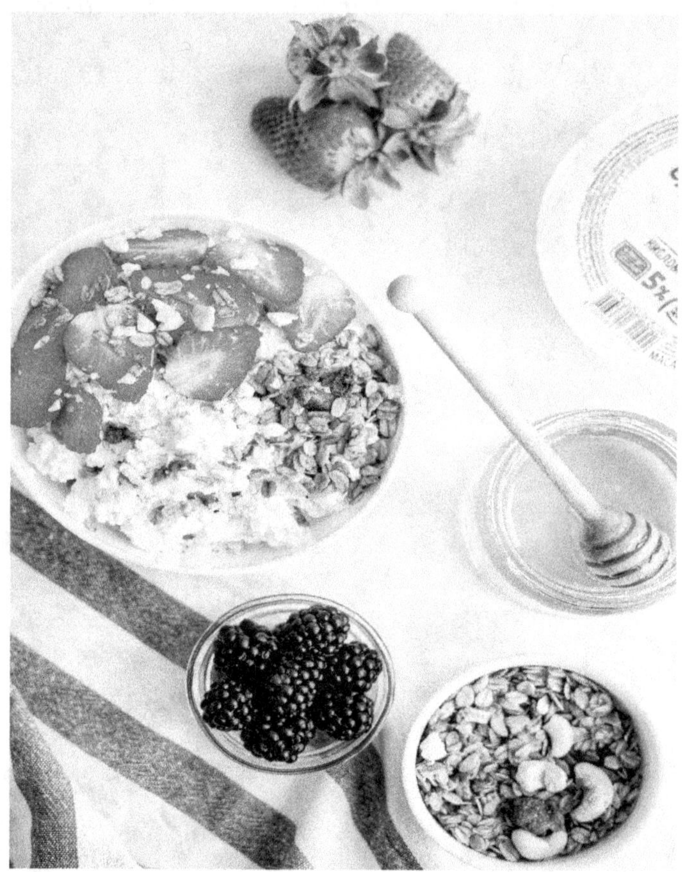

Make your own granola bar for breakfast or as a mid-morning snack. Homemade granola bars are another gritty option that you could have for breakfast and then take leftovers to snack on later. Grab your favorite oats, seeds, and nuts, combine with honey, butter, peanut butter, and brown sugar, and you've got the foundation for various kinds of granola bars.

Ingredients:

Cooking spray.

2 cups rolled oats.

1/2 cup shredded coconut.

½ cup honey

2 tablespoons of creamy peanut butter.

1 teaspoon of vanilla extract.

⅛ teaspoon salt.

How To Make Granola Bars

Granola bars are quite simple to make at home. The whole, step-by-step recipe is provided below, but here's a quick preview of what you may expect:

Prep Time: 15 minutes.

Cook Time: 25 minutes.

Total time: 1 hour and 40 minutes.

Serves: 8

- Get the oats and the coconut, then toast it in the oven.
- Combine the remaining ingredients over medium heat.
- Pour the peanut butter mixture over the coconut and toasted oats.
- Bake until the granola reaches your preferred texture.
- Let cool completely before cutting.

Instructions:

- Prepare your oven and preheat it at 325 degrees Fahrenheit (165 degrees Celsius).

- Grease a 9-inch-square baking dish.

- Spread the oats and coconut equally on a baking sheet.

- Toast the oats and coconut in a preheated oven for about 10 minutes before transferring to a large mixing bowl.

- In a saucepan, combine honey, peanut butter, vanilla, and salt over medium-low heat.

- Cook and stir until smooth. Pour the honey mixture over the oatmeal and coconut. Stir to coat.

- Carefully Spread the mixture evenly round in the baking dish you've prepared.

- Bake in a preheated oven until dry, about 15 minutes for crunchy granola bars and less if you prefer chewy. Cool fully before cutting.

Make it simple with some bread and a glass of milk.

If you get morning sickness, keeping things simple with toast is a good option. Bread has carbohydrates, which help to keep your energy levels up, and it's easy to snack on when you're not hungry. Spread with peanut butter or marmite and serve with a glass of milk for dairy.

Why is breakfast so vital during pregnancy

Breakfast is an essential element of any balanced diet, not only while pregnant. When you get up from a long (and ideally pleasant) night's sleep, your energy levels are low. As a result, you'll most likely be in need of an energy boost to provide your body with the fuel it requires to function properly. If you skip breakfast on a regular basis, you may find yourself inclined to snack on high-fat and sugar-containing foods between meals4, which will only deliver a short burst of energy rather than the slow-release energy you require to fuel your day.

However, some people have difficulty eating as soon as they get out of bed, which may be exacerbated during pregnancy. If this sounds familiar, consider starting the day with a small breakfast portion and letting your hunger grow gradually.

Eating breakfast in early pregnancy can be difficult if you suffer from morning sickness. Again, eat in little portions and stick to foods like dry wholemeal toast or crackers, which will supply you with energy while not being too harsh on your stomach.

CHAPTER 4: Energizing Lunches for Mom-to-Be

Advice on nourishing meals during pregnant Choose a midday meal that will provide you a sufficient amount of protein and fiber to keep you feeling full and energized.

Consider having a small smoothie for calcium, a salad for vitamins and fiber, and a whole grain bread sandwich for carbohydrates and protein. Add some healthy fat from almonds, avocado, or olive oil, and you have the makings of the ideal dinner.

Here are some additional pointers to remember:

Release the pressure: Don't make an effort to include every nutrient in your meal. There's still dinner and snacks to complete your day.

Quality over quantity: Overindulging in midday meals might make you feel drowsy and lethargic, which is something you may already experience when you don't eat. For additional energy, choose lean protein, whole grains, and produce over saturated fats and deep-fried foods.

Hydrate: Make sure you have a few 8-ounce glasses of water during lunchtime and a minimum of 10 glasses of water each day. It will lessen bloating and prevent bladder infections.

Lunchtime meals to stay away from

In addition to avoiding smoked seafood, undercooked eggs, and other breakfast items, pregnant women should avoid the following foods at lunch:

Lunch foods: Hot dogs, pâté, salami, bologna, and other deli meats may host listeria if not stored properly. In addition, a lot of them include preservatives and additives like nitrites, so for the time being, avoid packaged meats.

Certain fish and sushi: You can take up to 12 ounces of canned light tuna or salmon per week, but avoid foods high in methylmercury, such as shark, swordfish, king mackerel, and tilefish. The same is true for any kind of sushi that contains raw fish, as it might harbor bacteria.

Sugary yogurts: While a strawberry yogurt might seem healthy, many fruit-flavored yogurts include about the same amount of sugar as a tiny candy bar. Select low-fat, simple types and replace the fruit with your own sliced pieces.

Soft cheese: Don't eat lunch on chips and cheese dip. Steer clear of soft cheeses that may contain listeria, such as feta, blue cheese, Camembert, queso blanco, queso fresco, and brie.

Meat that is undercooked: Eat properly to feel well. To reduce your risk of upset stomach, avoid eating raw or undercooked meat and stick to well-cooked meat.

Women who eat well while they're expecting can minimize a host of pregnancy symptoms, including morning sickness and mood swings, and are more likely to deliver on time and have a speedier postpartum recovery. Now that's definitely easy to stomach!

Lunchtime meals to eat

Because this is the midday meal, when energy might be flagging, it's important to eat a variety of foods, including:

Salads: Filled with vitamins, minerals and fiber, salads make a perfect lunch. Boost the taste and nutritious value of a salad or grain bowl by adding some protein, like tuna, salmon, chicken, shrimp, beans or lentils. Make sure to skip the Caesar though, as that dressing typically contains raw eggs.

Soups: No matter the season, soups make a great midday meal. They can be as hearty as you want, can play well with others we're looking at you, sandwiches and can be filled with protein and fiber. Eat em' cold or eat em' hot and make a double batch, so you can freeze some for another time.

Sandwiches: Wraps, paninis, double-deckers no matter what type of sandwich you crave, make it a healthy one, with lean protein, fiber and whole grains. Fill it to the seams with greens so you optimize your lunch. Just forgo any sprouts, as they can harbor bacteria, and skip traditional lunch meats (more on that below!) for more creative solutions.

Smoothie bowls: The perfect vehicle for all things tastefully healthy, this meal can marry protein, calcium and vitamin-rich foods like yogurt, fruit, nuts and seeds, and whole grains, all in one gorgeous bowl.

Soups

Sunset Lentil and Sweet Potato Soup

This is as gratifying a soup as it gets: thick, full-bodied, and loaded with vegetables and flavorful lentils. You'll also be eating a lot of fiber and lots of nutrients. The best part is that you can make it once and then eat it repeatedly (you can freeze the extra and carry it in a thermos for lunch the next day).

This preparation is made even easier by the use of an immersion blender, which is a wand-shaped hand blender that you can insert directly into the pot. It will also come in handy for pureeing baby food in the upcoming months.

Ingredients:

- 1 tablespoon olive oil

- ½ chopped medium onion

- One large stalk of celery, cut thinly

- one chopped medium red bell pepper

- one cup of finely sliced carrots

- Two minced garlic cloves, if preferred

- One teaspoon of ground cumin

- 1/4 teaspoon ground coriander

- Two teaspoons of new thyme leaves

- Two cups of washed red or green lentils

- Two cans (14.5 oz, or roughly 4 cups) low-sodium chicken stock

- One can, weighing between 14 and 15 ounces chopped tomatoes

- One large or two small sweet potatoes, peeled and cut into ¾-inch cubes (approximately one pound total).

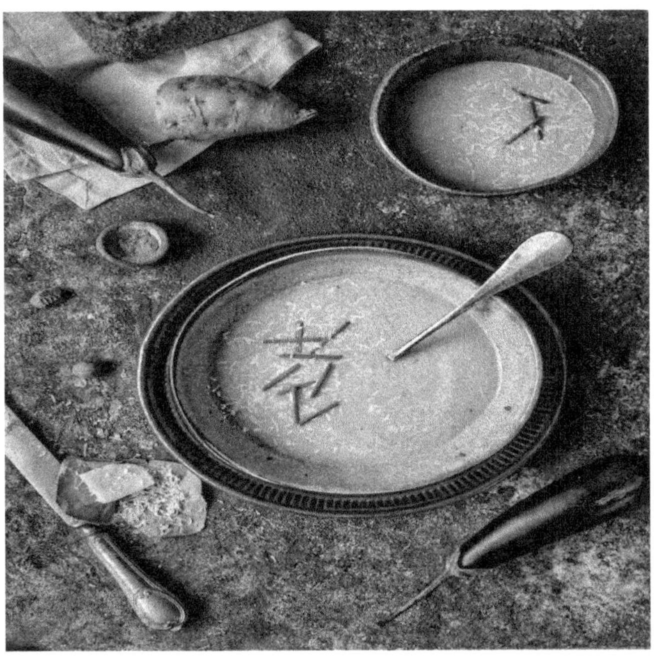

Guidelines:

- Heat up the oil in a big pot or 10-quart Dutch oven over medium heat.

- Add carrots, red pepper, onion, and celery.

- Cook, stirring, for 3 minutes.

- Add the thyme, coriander, cumin, and garlic. Cook, stirring frequently, until veggies are softened, about 10 minutes.

- Add the sweet potatoes, tomatoes, lentils, and broth.

- Bring to a boil, then lower the heat and simmer, stirring frequently, for 35 to 40 minutes, or until potatoes are tender.

- If necessary, add more water to the soup to get the right consistency.

- Half of the soup should be removed and pureed until smooth in a food processor, blender, or immersion blender.

- Return the purée to the pot and stir over low heat before serving.

Serves nine cups.

Information on Nutrition:

- One cup of food has 230 calories.

- Protein: half a serving

- Vitamin C: half a dish

- One serving of green or yellow vegetables

- Nearly two servings of whole grains

- Iron, fiber, and fat: some

Carrot-Ginger Soup

With the combination of sweet carrots and spicy (but calming) ginger, each cup of this velvety, filling soup packs a nutrient-dense punch. Best of all, it's ideal if you're really sensitive to smells since it doesn't need sautéing. (Appoint your companion to cut the onions for you.)

Ingredients:

- 1 sliced medium sweet onion

- One bag (16 ounces) young carrots

- 1 tablespoon freshly chopped ginger

- Four cups of low-sodium vegetable

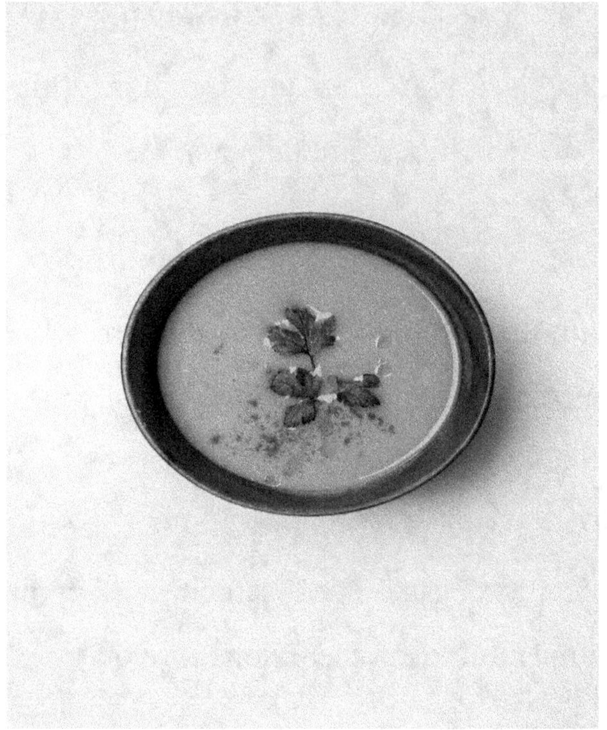

or chicken broth

- freshly squeezed lemon juice

- Black pepper with salt

- For garnish, 8 tablespoons plain low-fat yogurt

Guidelines:

- Ginger, carrots, and onion should all be combined in a big saucepan over medium-high heat. Pour in the broth.

- Boil, then lower the heat and cook the carrots until they are tender.

- Allow the soup to cool a little. If needed, transfer soup to a food processor or blender and purée in batches until smooth.

- Put soup back in the pot and reduce heat down to medium.

- Get salt, pepper, add them and lemon juice to taste.

- Cook until well heated.

- Transfer to a serving dish and place two teaspoons of yogurt on top of each.

4 servings

Information on Nutrition:
- Ninety calories per serving
- ½ serving of vitamin C
- Three portions of green or yellow veggies
- Extra veggies: half a serving

Garden Gazpacho

Although it requires some chopping, this midsummer soup blends quickly.

It only takes a minute to combine this refreshing and nutritious soup. Use deep red hothouse tomatoes or prepare this during the peak tomato season for maximum taste.

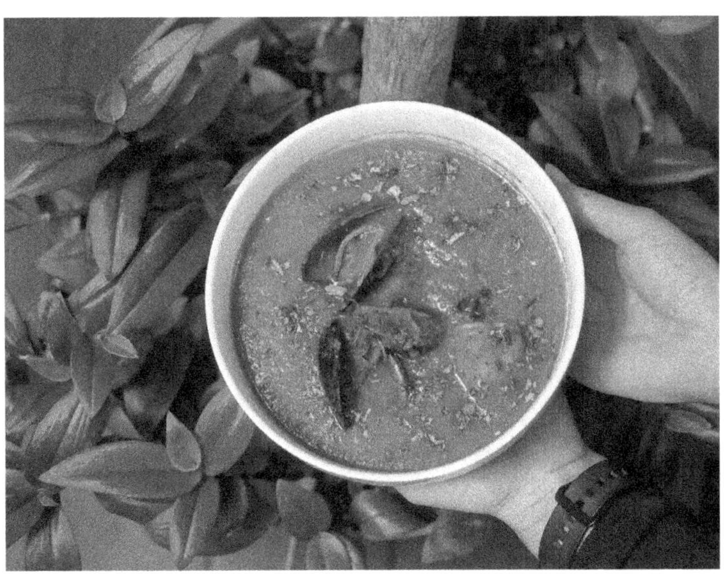

Ingredients:

- 3 quartered tomatoes
- two celery stalks, diced
- One chopped and seeded red bell pepper
- One peeled, seeded, and roughly chopped cucumber
- One little red onion, sliced into eighths after peeling
- One little clove of peeled and crushed garlic
- 1¼ cups of mixed vegetable juice
- Two tablespoons pure olive oil
- One tablespoon balsamic vinegar
- Add pepper and salt.
- one lime, thinly sliced

Guidelines:

- All ingredients except lime wedges should be combined in a food processor and pulsed until the mixture turns soupy but the vegetables are still slightly chunky.

- To get the finest flavor, chill soup for at least half an hour. Accompany with wedges of lime.

Yields roughly six servings.

Information on Nutrition:
- 95 calories in a cup of food
- Vitamin C: half a dish
- One dish of green or yellow vegetables
- One serving of other vegetable

Broccoli and Cheese Soup

Broccoli, cheese, and potatoes are old friends; this velvety smooth, vitamin-rich soup brings them together for a wonderful reunion. It's so delicious that you won't miss the cream — or the calories. To save time, use a package of broccoli florets.

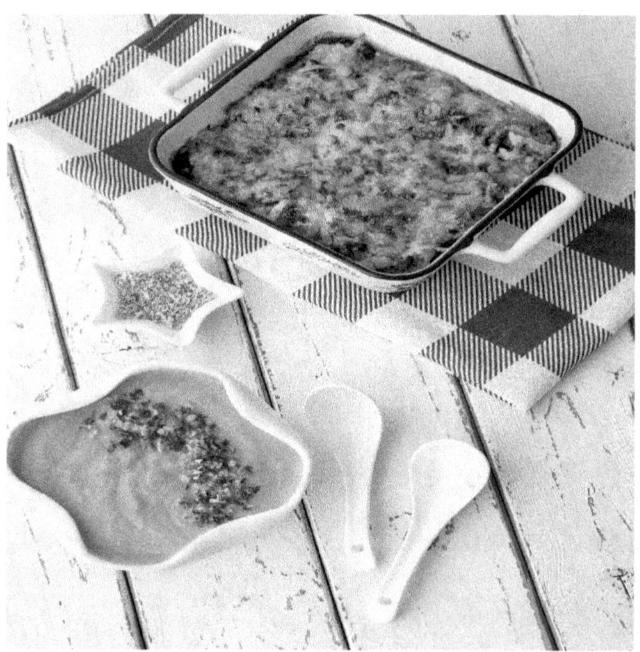

Ingredients:

- 1 tablespoon olive oil or butter.

- ½ medium onion, chopped

- 1 garlic clove, minced

- 2 cups broccoli florets

- 1 medium Yukon Gold potato, diced

- 2 ½ cups of low-sodium chicken or veggie broth.

- ¾ cup shredded cheddar cheese

- Add ¼ cup buttermilk or more to taste.

- Salt with Black pepper

Guideline:

- In a large saucepan set over medium heat, dissolve the butter.

- Cook for 5 minutes, or until the onion and garlic have softened.

- Turn the heat up to high and bring the broccoli, potato, and chicken broth to a boil.

- Reduce the heat, cover the saucepan, and simmer for about 7 minutes, or until the broccoli and potato are tender.

- Allow the broccoli combination to cool somewhat before transferring it to a blender or food processor. Puree the mixture until satiny smooth, working in batches if necessary.

- Return the soup to the saucepan, add ¼ cup of cheese and buttermilk.

- Cook the soup over low heat for about 3 minutes, or until the cheese melts. Add salt and pepper to taste.

- Pour the soup into serving bowls and sprinkle with the remaining 3 tablespoons of cheese.

Tip: If pregnancy indigestion is causing heartburn, try removing garlic and/or onion from your soups.

Serves 2

Nutritional Information: One serving provides:

- Protein: half a serving.
- Calcium: nearly two servings.
- Vitamin C: 2 servings.
- Green leafy and yellow veggies and fruits: 2 servings.

- Other fruits and vegetables: 1/2 serving
- Fat: ½ serving.

Roasted Butternut Squash and Apple Soup

Broccoli, cheese, and potatoes are old friends; this velvety smooth, vitamin-rich soup brings them together for a wonderful reunion. It's so delicious that you won't miss the cream — or the calories. To save time, use a package of broccoli florets.

Apple juice adds flavor to this seasonal soup.

The simplest approach to clean gritty leeks is to slice them thinly and then place them in a strainer under running water. Run your fingers through the slices, dividing the circles to remove dirt.

Tip: To make a less sweet soup, use chicken broth for the apple juice.

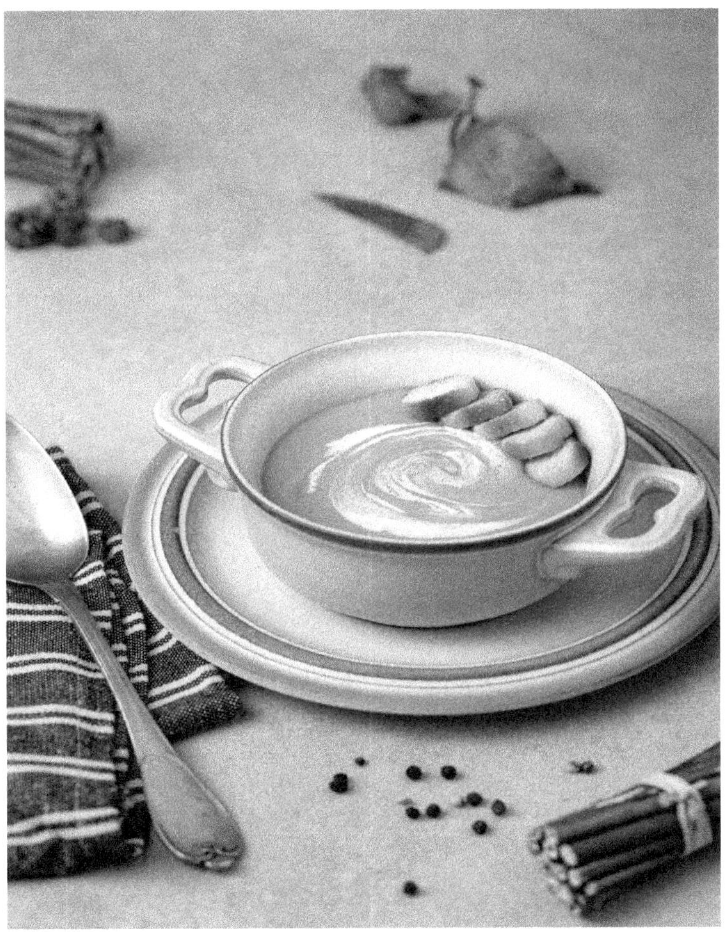

Ingredients:

- 1 Tbsp + 1 tsp olive oil.

- 1 2- lb butternut squash, halved lengthwise and planted.
- Salt and pepper.
- 2 leeks, cleaned and thinly sliced
- Ingredients: 1 chopped celery stalk, 1 peeled and sliced carrot, and 1/2 tsp fresh or 1/4 tsp dried thyme.
- 1 can (14½ oz). Chicken broth with low sodium
- 1/2 cup calcium-fortified apple juice or cider.
- 3/4 cup grated Parmesan cheese

Instructions:

- Preheat the oven to 375 F. With a parchment or foil, carefully line a rimmed baking sheet.

- Drizzle 1 tablespoon oil over the cut surfaces of the squash; season with salt and pepper.

- Place the squash, cut side down, on the set distance. Singe for 45 twinkles, or until tender.

- Meanwhile, heat 1 teaspoon of oil in a large nonstick saucepan over medium heat.

- Cook the leeks, celery, and carrot for 15 minutes, or until tender, stirring frequently. Transfer to the bowl of the food processor.

- Scrape squash into a processor with a large spoon, discarding the peel.

- Puree 1 cup of the broth until smooth. Return to the pot; add the apple juice and enough broth to thin to the desired consistency.

- Set on medium-low heat to warm through. Season to taste with salt and pepper.

- Garnish each plate with 2 tablespoons of Parmesan cheese.

Makes six servings.

Soup can be made two days ahead. Refrigerate, securely covered.

Nutritional Information:

- 1 cup serving is 140 calories.
- Calcium: 1/2 serving.

- Green/yellow vegetables: two servings
- Other vegetables: 1/2 serving.

Butternut Squash and Pear Soup

This bisque is fragrant and lovely, but it appears to have taken a lot of effort. Cooking is much easy and faster than you might imagine, and the nutritional benefits are substantial. And, most of all, the sweet and slightly spicy mix of squash and pears will satisfy your taste senses.

- 1 small butternut squash (approximately 1 ½ pounds), chopped.
- 3 cups low-sodium vegetable or chicken broth.
- Salt
- 1 tablespoon butter or canola oil.
- One small onion, very thinly sliced
- Two red pears, peeled, cored, and finely chopped
- 1 ½ teaspoon curry powder.

- ¾ teaspoon ground turmeric.

- 1/2 teaspoon ground ginger (optional)

- 1/3 cup plain, whole-milk yogurt

- White Pepper

- 1/2 cup finely shredded cheddar cheese.

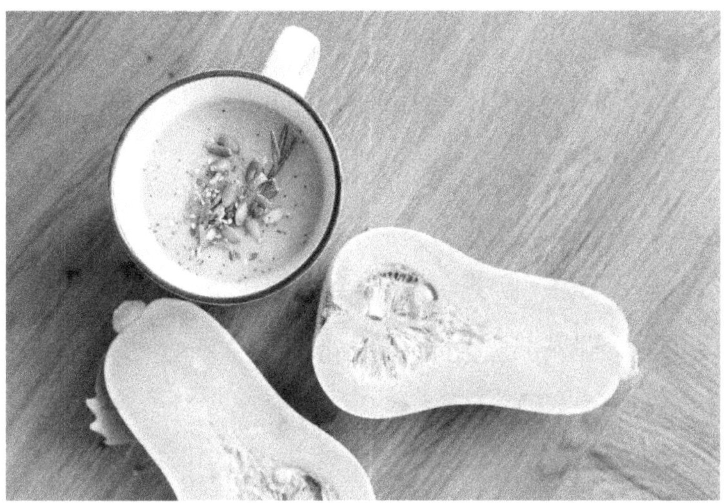

Direction:

- In a large saucepan over medium-high heat, bring the squash, 2 ½ cups vegetable broth, and a pinch of salt to a boil.

- Reduce the heat and simmer for approximately 35 minutes, or until the squash softens.

- Set the squash and boiling liquid aside.

- While the squash is cooking, melt the butter in a large skillet set over medium heat.

- Cook the onion, turning regularly, until softened, about 5 minutes.

- Cook the pears, stirring regularly, until softened, about 5 minutes. Bring the curry powder, turmeric, and ginger (if using) to a simmer with the remaining ½ cup vegetable broth.

- Cover the skillet and heat for 10 minutes, or until the flavors mix.

- Combine the onion and pear combination with the cooked squash. Allow the squash mixture to cool somewhat before transferring it to a blender or food processor, working in batches if required, to purée until smooth.

- Return the soup to the pot, mix in the yogurt, and season to taste with salt and pepper. Place the saucepan over low heat and let the soup cook through, 2 to 3 minutes.

- Don't let it boil. Pour the soup into serving bowls and top with 2 tablespoons cheddar cheese.

Serves 4

Tip: Only serving two (and a half) people for dinner tonight. Make this soup to step 3, then divide in half. Step 4: Combine 3 tablespoons of yogurt and ¼ cup of cheddar cheese. The remaining soup can be refrigerated, covered, for up to two days. Reheat it before proceeding to step 4.

Nutritional Information:

- 1 piece (1 bowl) offers:
- Calcium: 1/2 serving.
- Green leafy and yellow veggies and fruits: two servings.
- Other fruits and vegetables: one serving.

Roasted Vegetable Soup

This soup is rich and thick, full of fall veggies and vitamins, yet contains no cream or butter. Roasting the vegetables takes less than an hour and yields a beautifully nuanced flavor.

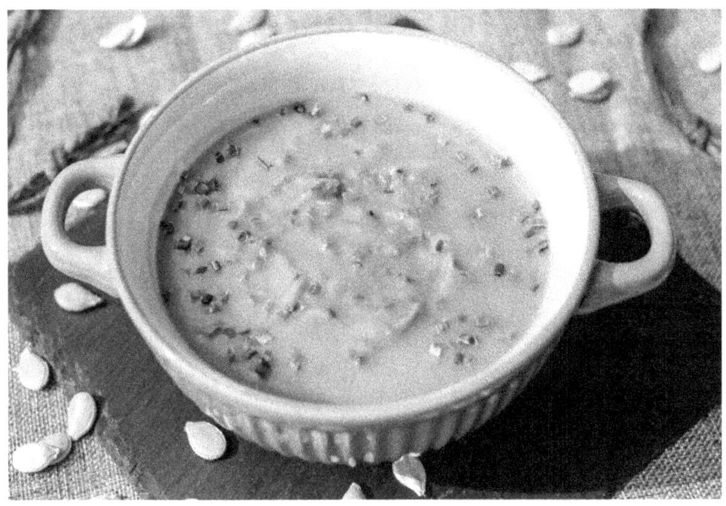

- Cooking oil spray
- 2 medium-sized carrots sliced into 1-inch cubes (about 1 ½ cups)
- 2 medium-sized parsnips, sliced into 1-inch slices (approximately one cup)

- One small rutabaga, chopped into 1-inch cubes (approximately 1 cup).
- 1 small red onion, quartered, then sliced in half.
- 1 tablespoon of olive oil.
- Salt and black pepper.
- 4 teaspoons of fresh thyme leaves.
- 3–4 cups chicken broth
- Toasted Pumpkin Seeds
- Chopped fresh flat-leafed parsley

Direction:

- Preheat the onion to 400 degrees Fahrenheit. Spray a large, rimmed baking sheet with cooking oil spray.

- In a large bowl, combine the carrots, parsnips, rutabaga, and onion; drizzle with olive oil and toss to coat evenly.

- Place the vegetable mixture in an equal layer on the prepared baking sheet.

- Sprinkle salt, pepper, and 3 tablespoons of thyme leaves over top.

- Bake until the vegetables are soft, about 45 minutes, stirring periodically.

- In a large saucepan, combine roasted veggies, 3 cups chicken broth, and remaining 1 ½ teaspoons thyme leaves.

- Bring to a boil over high fire, then decrease heat and simmer until very soft, about 15 minutes.

- Let the soup cool somewhat, then working in stages if required, transfer it to a blender or food processor and purée it until slightly lumpy or smooth (as you choose). If the soup appears to be too thick, gradually add some chicken broth to lighten it. Check for seasoning, and add additional salt and/or pepper as needed.

- If the soup has cooled too much, transfer it back to the saucepan and gradually reheat over low heat.

- Sprinkle pumpkin seeds and parsley over top immediately before serving. The soup can be refrigerated and covered for up to two days.

Serves 4

Nutritional Information:
- 1 piece (1 bowl) offers:
- Green leafy and yellow veggies and fruits: one serving.
- Other fruits and vegetables: one serving.

Tomato Soup With Avocado

This adaptable soup is wonderful hot or chilled, and is packed with flavor and nutrition.

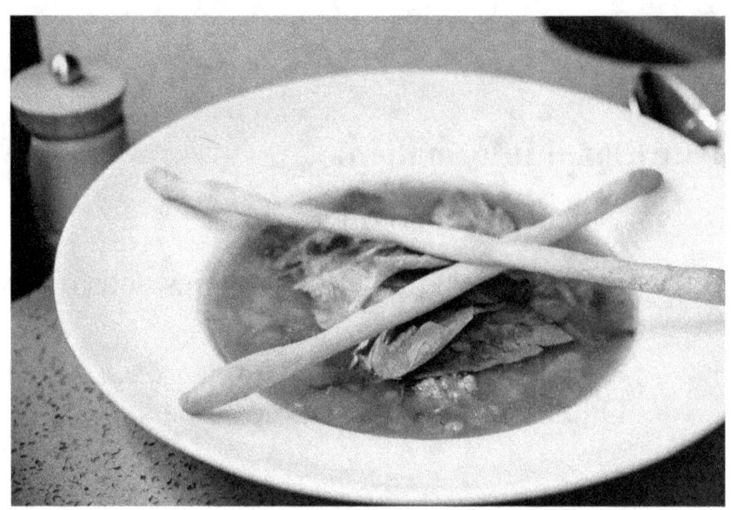

Ingredients:

- 2 teaspoons of olive oil.

- Three scallions, both white and light green, clipped and thinly sliced

- ½ teaspoon of roughly chopped garlic (from one clove)

- Use 4 medium-sized ripe tomatoes, seeded and coarsely chopped, or 1 ½ cups canned crushed tomatoes with juices.

- 4 cups of tomato juice or vegetable juice (such as V8)

- 2 tablespoons dried basil or ¼ cup finely sliced fresh basil leaves.

- Salt and black pepper.

- Diced avocado for serving.

- For serving, coarsely cut 1/2 red bell pepper.

- 4 lime wedges for serving.

Direction:

- In a saucepan, warm the olive oil over medium heat. Cook the scallions and garlic for about 2 minutes, or until softened.

- Bring the tomatoes, tomato juice, and basil to a boil over medium-high heat. Reduce the heat and let the soup simmer for 15 minutes, or until the flavors are fully mixed. Season to taste with salt and pepper.

- Pour the soup into bowls, top with avocado and bell pepper, and serve with lime wedges. The soup can also be cooled. It can be kept refrigerated, covered, for up to two days.

Serves 4

Nutrition information: One portion (1 dish) contains:

- Vitamin C: 2 ½ servings with tomato juice, 3 with vegetable juice.
- Consume 1 ½ servings of green leafy and yellow vegetables and fruits, preferably in vegetable juice.

Sandwiches

Classic Egg Salad

A comfort-food staple that you'll make for your kids in a few years. Research has shown that red onions have a milder flavor than white or even the yellow onions. (You can also omit the onion completely.)

Tip: For added calcium, add cheese slices to your sandwich.

Ingredients:
- Three big eggs.
- 2 tablespoons plain yogurt.
- 1 tablespoon mayonnaise.
- 1 teaspoon fresh lemon juice
- ½ teaspoon Dijon mustard.
- 1/2 cup quartered cherry tomatoes.

- ½ celery stalk, minced (approximately ¼ cup).

- 1 tablespoon minced red onion

- 2 teaspoons chopped fresh dill, if desired

- Salt and pepper.

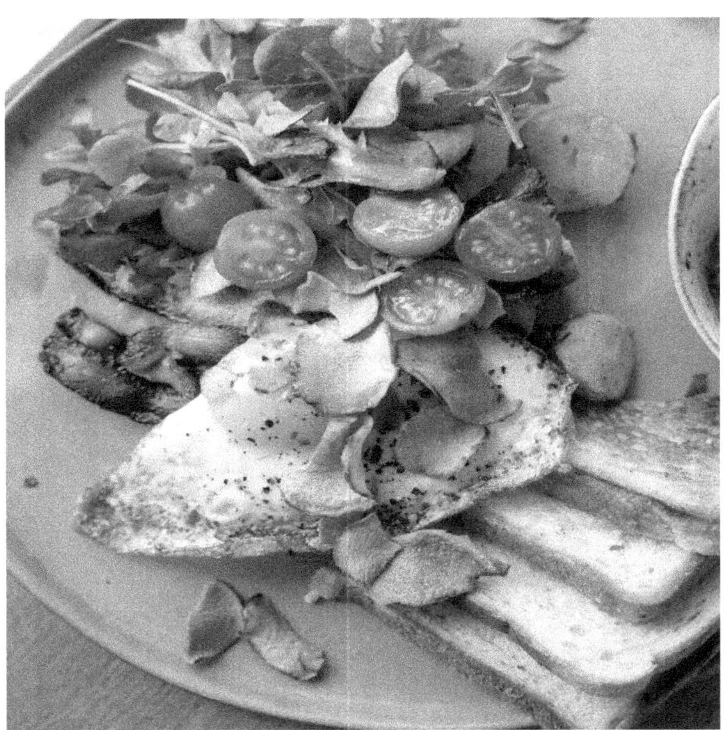

Instructions:

- Get the eggs and Place them in a medium saucepan and cover it with water.

- Bring to a boil on high heat. Remove pan from heat, cover, and let stand for 10 minutes. Drain eggs and rinse with cool water. Peel and chop.

- Meanwhile, in a medium bowl, add yogurt, mayonnaise, lemon juice, and mustard. Fold in egg, tomatoes, celery, onion, and dill. Season with salt and pepper if required.

Makes 1½ cups (enough to fill one large sandwich).

Make ahead: The salad can be prepared up to one day in advance. Refrigerate, securely covered.

Nutritional Information:

- 1 serving is 285 calories.
- Protein: One serving.
- Vitamin C: one serving.
- Green/yellow vegetable: 1/2 serving.
- Other vegetables: 1/2 serving.
- Fat: 1 serving.
- Iron: Some.

Classic Egg Salad Sandwich With Cheese

Ingredients:
- Three huge eggs.
- 2 tablespoons plain yogurt.
- 1 tablespoon mayonnaise.
- 1 teaspoon fresh lemon juice

- ½ teaspoon Dijon mustard.

- 1/2 cup quartered cherry tomatoes.

- ½ celery stalk, minced (approximately ¼ cup).

- 1 tablespoon minced red onion

- 2 teaspoons chopped fresh dill, if desired

- Salt and pepper.

- 2 slices whole wheat bread.

- 1 slice of reduced-fat cheese.

- Lettuce

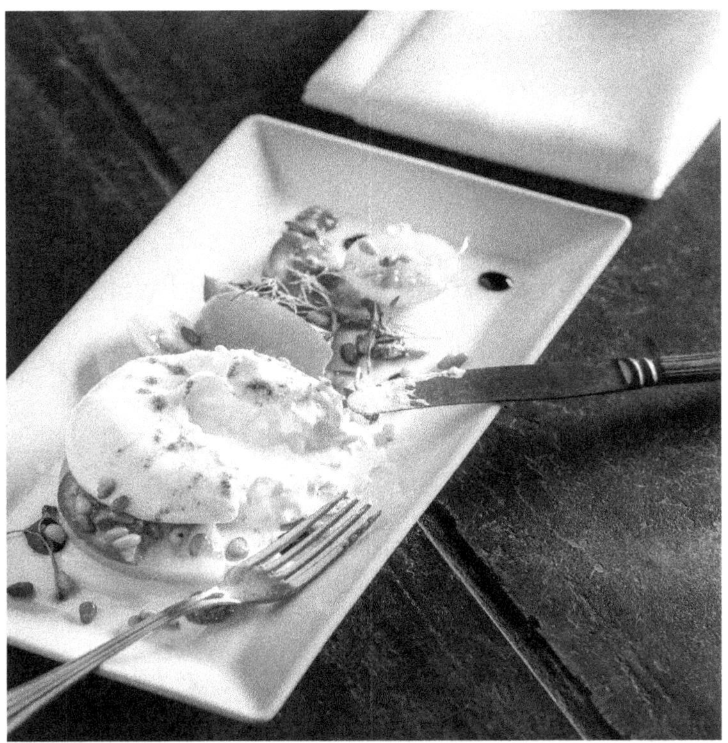

Instructions:

- Get a medium saucepan and put the eggs inside, then cover with water.

- Bring to a boil on high heat. Remove pan from heat, cover, and let stand for 10 minutes.

- Drain eggs and rinse with cool water. Peel and chop.

- Meanwhile, in a medium bowl, add yogurt, mayonnaise, lemon juice, and mustard.

- Fold in egg, tomatoes, celery, onion, and dill. Season with salt and pepper if required.

- Serve on two slices of whole wheat bread, topped with a slice of reduced-fat cheese.

Makes 1½ cups (enough to fill one large sandwich).

Make ahead: The salad can be prepared up to one day in advance. Refrigerate, securely covered.

Nutritional Information:

- 1 sandwich equals 565 calories.
- Protein: One serving.
- Vitamin C: one serving.
- Calcium: One serving.
- Green/yellow vegetable: 1/2 serving.
- Other vegetables: 1/2 serving.
- Other fruit: one serving.
- Fat: 1 serving.
- Whole grains: two servings.
- Iron: Some.

Mediterranean Salmon Salad Sandwich

Canned salmon contains the same nutrients as fresh salmon but has a softer flavor.

Ingredients:

- 2 tablespoons plain yogurt.
- 1 tablespoon mayonnaise.
- 1 tablespoon fresh lemon juice
- 1 canned (7 ½ ounce) pink salmon, drained
- 1/2 cup drained white beans.
- 1/2 cup quartered cherry tomatoes.
- Small red bell pepper, seeded and diced into medium pieces.
- 2 tablespoons minced fresh basil leaves.
- Salt and pepper.
- Baby spinach leaves or salad greens

- 1 large whole wheat pita.

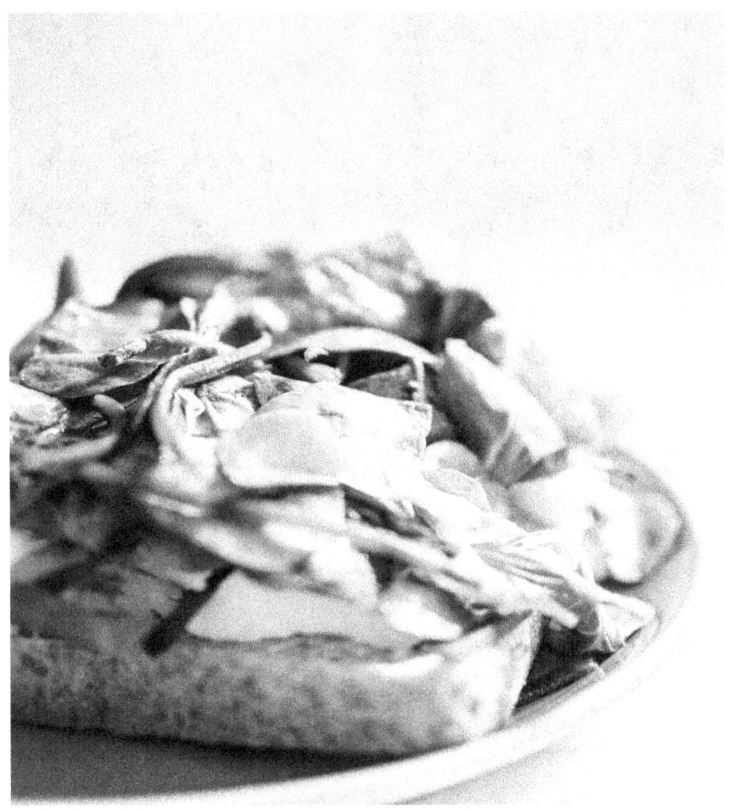

Instructions:

- In a medium bowl, combine yogurt, mayonnaise, and lemon juice.

- Fold in the fish, beans, tomatoes, bell peppers, and basil.

- Season with salt and pepper to taste. Stuff into pita pockets with veggies.

Make enough salad for two sandwiches.

Make ahead: The sandwich can be made up to one day in advance. Refrigerate, securely covered.

Nutritional Information:
- 1 serving equals 405 calories.
- Protein: One serving.
- Vitamin C: one serving.
- Calcium: One serving.
- Green/yellow vegetables: one serving
- Whole grains: two servings.

- Fat: 1/2 serving

Turkey Swiss Wrap

Experiment with the various types of hummus available; however, avoid garlic-flavored hummus if it affects your stomach.

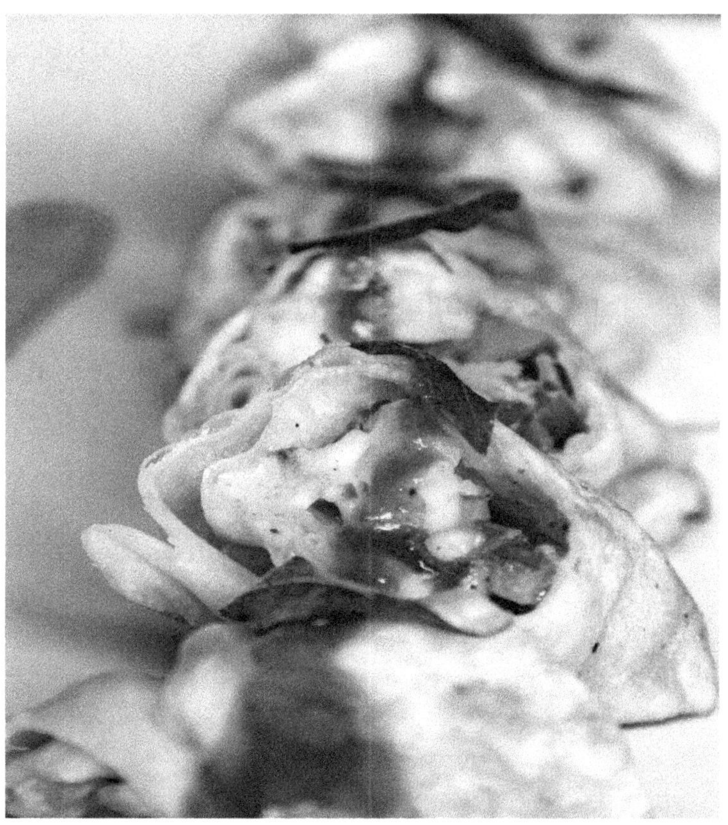

Ingredients:

- 1 tbsp prepared hummus.

- 1 large whole wheat tortilla.

- 4 oz cooked turkey, ½ ripe medium avocado, cut, and ½ cup baby spinach leaves.

- 2 tablespoons shredded Swiss or Jarlsberg cheese.

Instructions:

- Spread hummus over the tortilla. Layer turkey, avocado, spinach, and cheese on a tortilla.

- Roll up the sandwich. If packing to go, wrap it tightly with plastic wrap.

Make one sandwich.

Nutritional Information:

- 1 serving equals 530 calories.

- Protein: One serving.

- Calcium: 1/2 serving.

- Green/yellow vegetable: 1/2 serving.

- Other vegetables: one serving.

- Whole grains: two servings.

Chicken Caesar Salad Sandwich

Tip: Use leftover chicken for the sandwich filling, or buy a rotisserie chicken from the store.

Ingredients:

- 4 ounces (approximately one) cooked chicken breast, shredded or diced.

- 1 cup shredded romaine, 1/4 medium red bell pepper, seeded and finely sliced.

- 1/2 cup halved cherry tomatoes.

- 2 tablespoons grated Parmesan cheese.

- 1 tablespoon premade Caesar salad dressing.
- 2 tablespoons fresh lemon juice
- 1 large whole wheat pita.

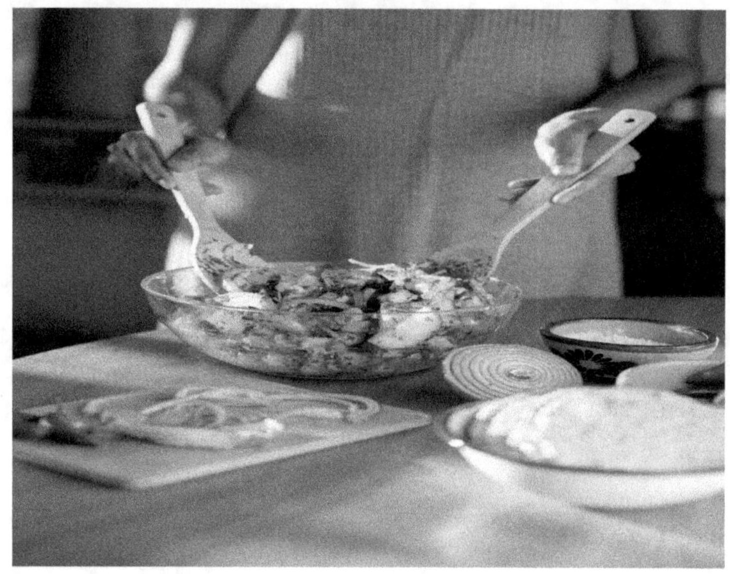

Instructions:

- In a medium bowl, combine all ingredients except the pita.

- Trim ½ inch off one edge of the pita and fill with salad. If you're creating a sandwich to go, cover it tightly in plastic wrap.

Make one sandwich.

Nutritional Information:
- 1 serving is 485 calories.
- Protein: One serving.
- Vitamin C: two servings.
- Calcium: 1/2 serving.
- Green/yellow vegetables: 1½ servings.
- Whole grains: two servings.
- Fat: 1 serving.

Lemon-Chicken Salad Sandwich

Serve three-quarters cup chicken salad with cheese, walnuts, and lettuce on two slices of whole wheat bread.

Ingredients:

- 2 boneless, skinless chicken breast halves with tenders removed (about 5 oz each).
- 1/4 cup low-fat yogurt
- 2 tablespoons mayonnaise.
- 1 tablespoon fresh lemon juice
- 1 teaspoon Dijon mustard.
- 1 medium stalk celery, thinly cut.
- 2 tablespoons coarsely sliced red onion.
- 1 tablespoon freshly chopped fresh tarragon.
- Salt and pepper.
- ¼ cup chopped walnuts

- 2 slices whole wheat bread.

- 1 deli slice cheese of your choosing

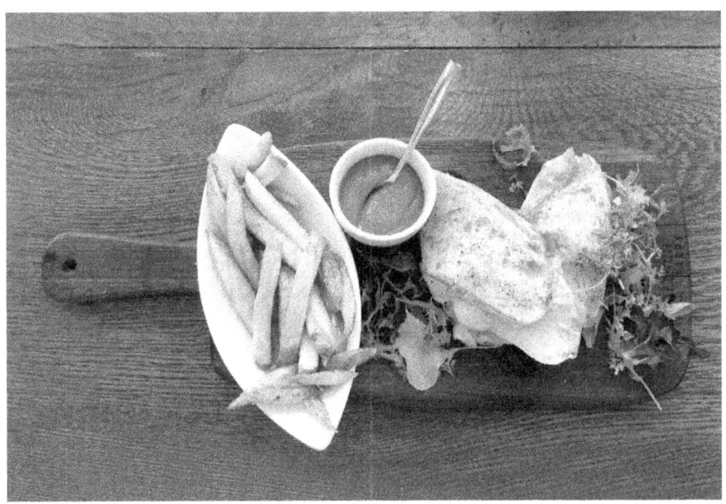

Instructions:

- Place the chicken breasts in a medium saucepan with enough water to cover. Place over high heat and come to a boil.

- Skim away any scum that forms. Reduce heat and simmer for 10 minutes.

- Remove pan from heat and let chicken cool in cooking liquid for 45 minutes.

- In a medium bowl, combine the yogurt, mayonnaise, lemon juice, and mustard. Shred the chicken into bite-sized pieces and combine with the celery, onion, and tarragon.

- Season with salt and pepper. Sprinkle with walnuts.

Make two cups. Serve in a 3/4-cup quantity on a sandwich and top with cheese.

Make ahead: The salad can be prepared up to one day in advance. Refrigerate, securely covered.

Nutritional Information:

- 1 sandwich equals 590 calories.

- Protein: One serving.

- Calcium: One or more servings

- Green leafy or yellow: 1/2 serving.

- Whole grains: two servings.

- Fat: 1 serving.

Wrap 'n' Roll

Toss cabbage, red bell pepper, tomato, Kalamata olives, and cheddar cheese with turkey or chicken (the ideal location for leftovers from the night before), then wrap it all up and you're ready to go.

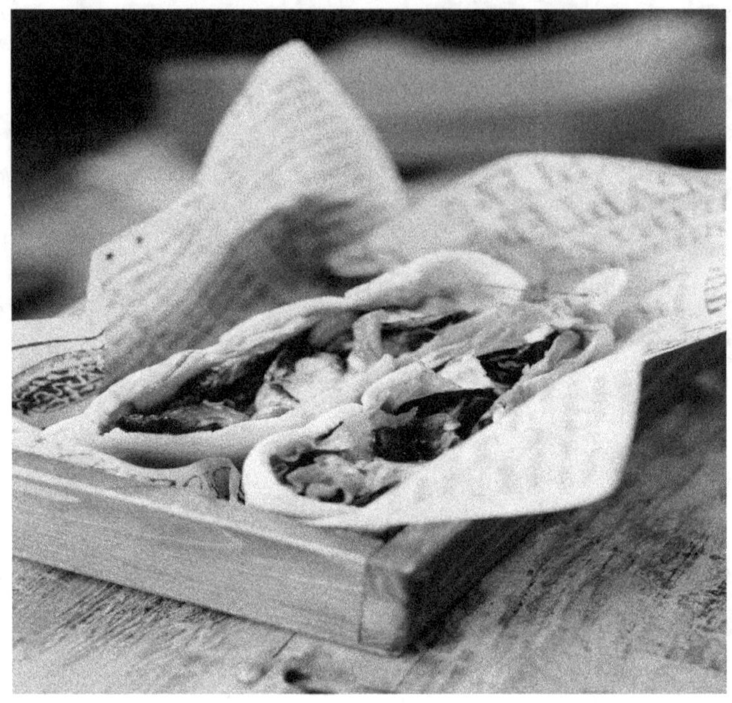

Ingredients:

- 1 tablespoon of olive oil.

- 1 tablespoon fresh lemon juice or seasoned rice vinegar.

- 1/8 teaspoon of dried oregano.

- Salt and black pepper.

- 1/2 cup coleslaw mix.

- Chop 1 plum tomato and dice 1/4 medium-sized red bell pepper.

- Chop 4 pitted Kalamata olives and 1/4 cup cubed cheddar cheese.

- One whole wheat tortilla or a seasoned wrap (12" diameter)

- 3 slices cooked turkey or chicken (about. 3 ounces).

Direction:

- Place the olive oil, lemon juice, and oregano in a mixing bowl and whisk to combine. Season to taste with salt and pepper.

- Toss together the coleslaw mix, tomato, bell pepper, olives, and cheese.

- Get and place the tortilla flat, gently on the work surface. Arrange the turkey on top, then ladle the salad into the center.

- Carefully and gradually Fold the sides of the tortilla over the filling. If you're taking the sandwich to go, cover it tightly in plastic wrap.

Make one sandwich.

Tip:

No wrap in sight? Use a whole wheat pita pocket instead. Trim ½ inch off one side of the pita and insert it into the bottom. Fill the pita with turkey slices, then add the salad. Wrap the sandwich tightly in plastic wrap before packing it for travel.

Nutritional Information: One section provides:

- Protein: One serving.
- Calcium: One serving.
- Vitamin C: two servings.
- Green leafy and yellow veggies and fruits: one serving.
- Whole grains and legumes: two servings.
- Fat: 1 serving.

A Better BLT

Here's a wonderful way to get your BLT fix without the calories while still getting enough of flavor, thanks to the mayo substitution - a white bean spread — that adds a delectable fifth dimension to the avocado, tomato, arugula, and veggie "bacon."

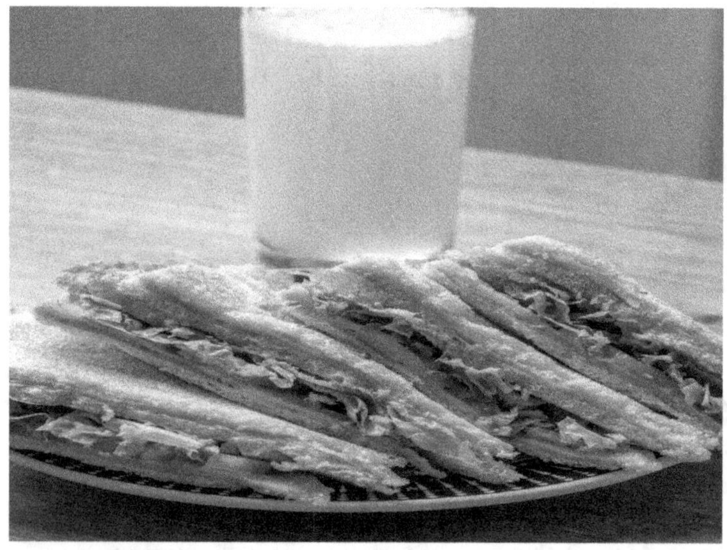

Ingredients:

- One whole grain roll.

- Two tablespoons (or more). White bean sandwich spread (recipe below)
- 1/2 cup arugula, watercress, or shredded red leaf lettuce with thick stems removed.
- ¼ cup grated carrot
- Cook 4 slices of vegetarian "bacon" (about 4 ounces) and slice 1/2 of a medium-sized avocado (ideally Hass).
- One plum tomato, sliced

Direction:

- sliced the roll in half, then spread the bean spread on both sliced sides.

- Layer the arugula, carrot, "bacon," avocado, and tomato on one side of the bun before topping with the other. If you're taking the sandwich to go, cover it tightly in plastic wrap.

Make one sandwich.

Nutritional information: One serving provides:

- Protein: 1/2 serving.
- Vitamin C: 1/2 serving if prepared with watercress.
- 1 ½ servings of green leafy vegetables and yellow fruits.
- Other fruits and vegetables: one serving.
- Whole grains and legumes: two servings.

White Bean Sandwich Spread

Use this creamy spread instead of mayonnaise on your sandwiches. Makes an excellent dip for crudités and pita strips.

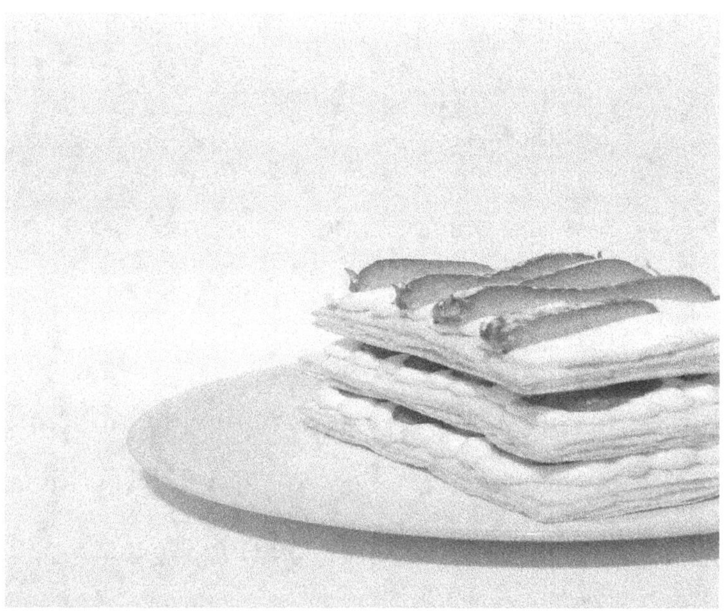

Ingredients:

- 2 tablespoons of olive oil.

- 1 huge clove of garlic, peeled and smashed.

- 1 can (approximately 15 ounces) of cannellini or Great Northern beans, rinsed and drained

- 2 tablespoons roughly chopped fresh cilantro or flat-leafed parsley
- Juice from 1 big lemon
- Salt and black pepper.

Direction:

- In a food processor, combine the olive oil, garlic, beans, cilantro, and lemon juice. Puree until smooth. Season to taste with salt and pepper.

- Serve at room temperature, warm in the microwave, or on the stovetop. The bean spread can be refrigerated and covered for up to 5 days.

Makes approximately 1 cup.

Tip: To make a hotter spread, replace chickpeas for the beans and add a teaspoon of ground toasted cumin seeds, as well as a dash of hot paprika and/or cayenne pepper. You can also add extra garlic.

Nutritional Information: One serving (¼ cup) provides:

- Whole grains and legumes: 1/2 serving.
- Iron comes from the beans.
- Fat: 1/2 serving

Salads and crudites

Salad with a Taco

This taco salad is exceptionally lean, in contrast to others, which have an astronomically high fat and calorie content. Fortunately, this recipe is just as delicious as the high-fat ones without having as many calories.

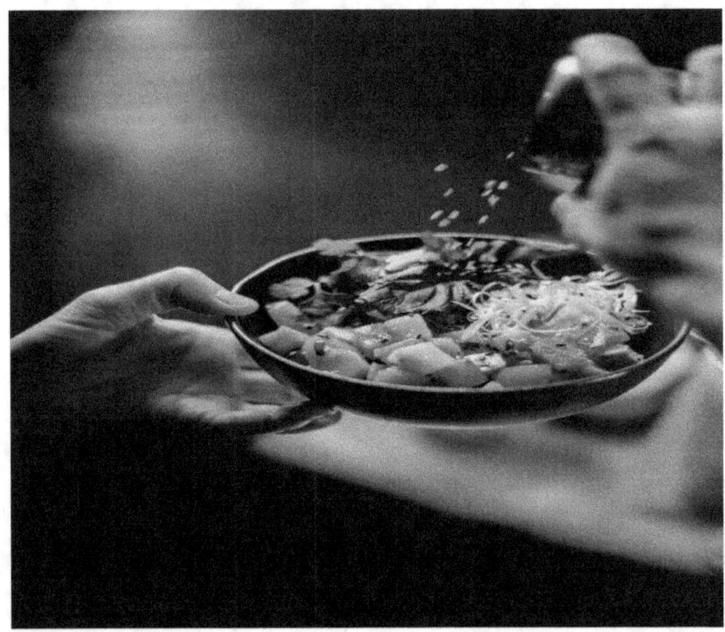

Ingredients:

- One tablespoon of olive oil

- two minced garlic cloves

- Eight ounces of lean ground beef, buffalo, or turkey breast; one medium red bell pepper; one medium yellow bell pepper; and one small onion; all diced.

- two tsp of chili powder

- One teaspoon of cumin powder

- ½ cup washed and well-drained canned kidney or pinto beans

- One and a half cups made salsa with tomatoes

- Two teaspoons of freshly chopped cilantro, optional

- Sauce from Tabasco (optional)

- Four cups of romaine lettuce, shredded

- Two big plum tomatoes, sliced and seeded

- Half a cup of shredded Monterey Jack or cheddar cheese
- ½ cup of cooked taco chips, slightly crumbled

Direction:

- In a big skillet, warm the olive oil over medium heat. Add the onion, bell peppers, and garlic; simmer for about 5 minutes, or until the ingredients are tender.

- Add the beef, cumin, and chili powder. Cook, stirring constantly, for 3 to 4 minutes, or until the meat is crumbly and cooked through.

- After adding the beans and salsa, raise the heat to a boil, lower it, and simmer for two minutes, or until the beans are thoroughly heated and the flavors are melded. Add the Tabasco, if using, and the cilantro.

- Place half of the beef mixture on top of each bed of lettuce after dividing the lettuce between two big plates or bowls. Divide the half of the chopped cheese and tomato among each salad, then top with ¼ cup of tortilla chips and serve right away.

Yields Two

Nutrition Information: One serving offers:

- 1 ½ servings of protein
- Calcium: One portion
- Four servings of vitamin C
- Three servings of yellow and green leafy vegetables and fruits

- Legumes and whole grains: ½ serving
- Iron: if the ground beef or buffalo is used
- Fat: half a serving

Tzatziki

Serve as a delicious sauce for grilled fish, a zesty spread over a sandwich or in a salad, or a tart dip for pita chips or vegetables. Peeling is not necessary for any sort of cucumber, but if you can get an English seedless cucumber, you will save time by not having to seed it.

Ingredients:

- 1 medium-sized grated and seeded cucumber
- 1 cup of low-fat plain yogurt
- One tablespoon of freshly squeezed lemon juice

- One little clove of minced garlic, if preferred
- One tablespoon of finely chopped fresh tarragon or dill
- Add salt to taste.

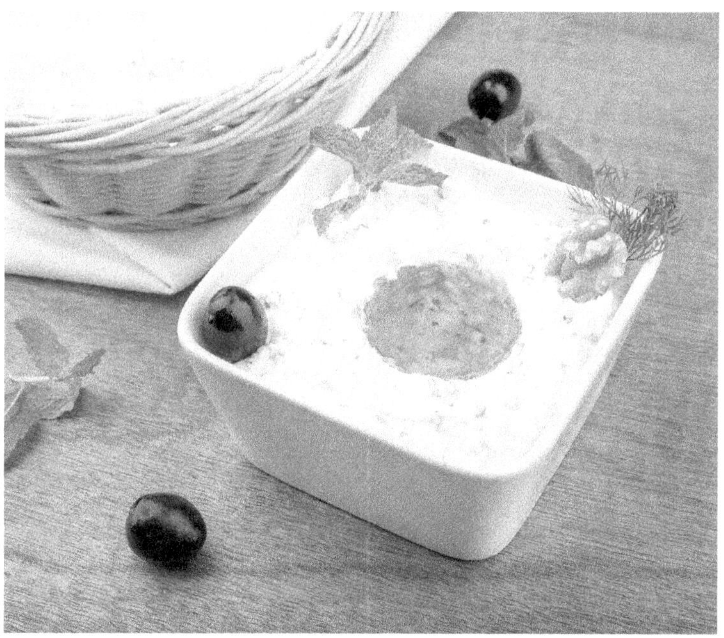

Guidelines:

- Using a kitchen towel, wrap the grated cucumber and squeeze dry. Mix the yogurt, dill, garlic, and lemon juice in a small bowl.

- Mix in the cucumber to coat. For one hour or up to twenty-four hours, cover and chill. If preferred, season with salt right before serving. Present chilled.

Plan ahead: Keep Tzatziki in the fridge for five days, securely covered.

Yields a pint.

Information about Nutrition:
- 30 calories in a ½-cup portion.
- Calcium: half a serving

Tzatziki with Peppers and Carrots

If you can find an English cucumber without seeds, use it; you won't have to spend time seeding it. Peeling the cucumber is not necessary, regardless of the variety used.

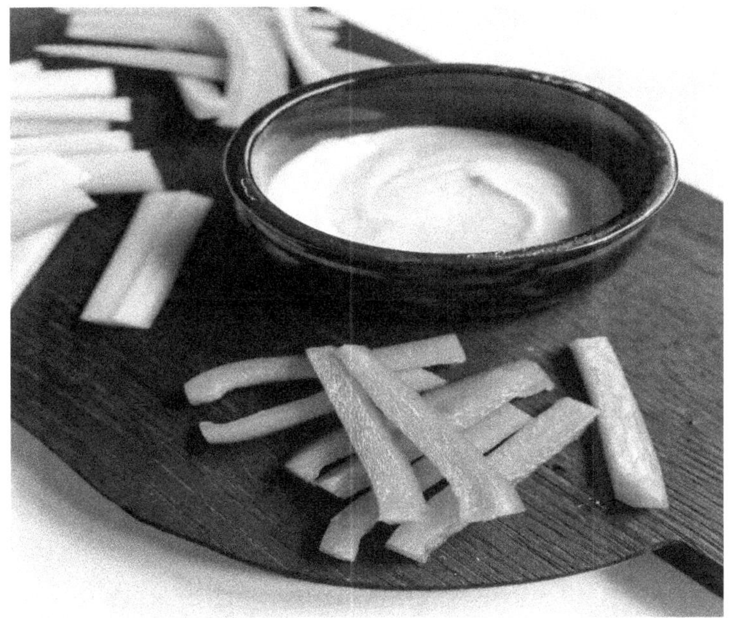

Ingredients:

- 1 medium-sized grated and seeded cucumber

- 1 cup of low-fat plain yogurt

- One tablespoon of freshly squeezed lemon juice

- One little clove of minced garlic, if preferred

- One tablespoon of finely chopped fresh tarragon or dill

- Add salt to taste.

- One cup of carrots and peppers

Guidelines:

- Using a kitchen towel, wrap the grated cucumber and squeeze dry.

- Combine yogurt, dill, garlic, and lemon juice in a small bowl. Add the cucumber and mix to coat. For one hour or up to twenty-four hours, cover and chill. If preferred, season with salt right before serving. Serve cold, dipping carrots and peppers, and savor!

Yields a pint of Tzatziki. A serving consists of ½ cup Tzatziki and 1 cup carrots and peppers.

Plan ahead: Keep Tzatziki in the fridge for five days, securely covered.

Information on Nutrition:
- 140 calories in one serving.
- Calcium: half a serving
- One serving of vitamin C
- Leafy greens or yellow: half a dish

Arugula Salad With Mango and Cucumber

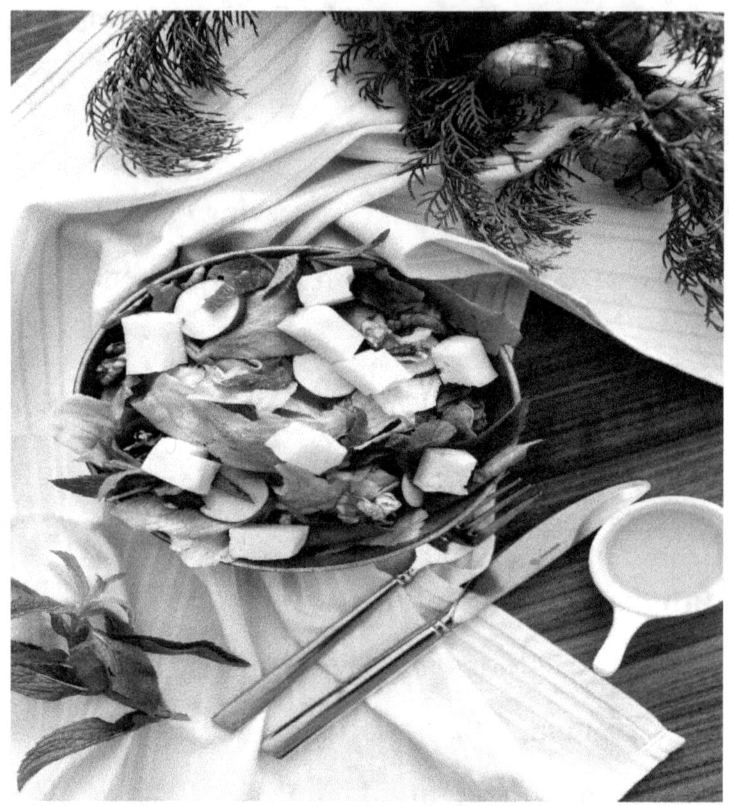

If mango is not in season or the arugula appears weary, try watercress and pear, spinach and apple, or…it's up to you!

Ingredients:

- 1 bunch of cleaned arugula (about 4 ounces).
- 1/2 mango, peeled and chopped.
- 1/2 large cucumber, peeled, seeded, and chopped.
- 2 to 3 tablespoons dressing of your choice.
- 2 tablespoons chopped fresh mint, if desired

Instructions:

- In a large serving bowl, combine the arugula, mango, and cucumber.
- Toss the salad with the dressing. Garnish portions with mint if desired.

Make two servings.

Nutritional Information:

- 1 serving is 125 calories.
- Vitamin C: 1/2 serving.
- Green/yellow vegetables: two servings
- Other vegetables: 1/2 serving.
- Fat: 1/2 serving

Wheat Berry Primavera

Are you tired of brown rice? Try Wheat Berry Primavera. Introduce chewy, nutty wheat berries to your whole grain diet. With crisp asparagus and a hint of tarragon, they add a unique twist to this classic springtime salute. No asparagus in sight? Swap in snap peas or frozen peas. Just make sure to sauté all of the vegetables until they are tender crisp. The salad can be served warm or at room temperature.

Ingredients:

- 2 cups plus ½ cup of reduced-sodium chicken broth, divided.

- ½ cup wheat berries

- 1 tablespoon plus 1 teaspoon extra virgin olive oil

- 1 medium shallot, minced 4 ounces (about 1/2 bunch) Trim asparagus ends and thinly slice. Chop ¼ medium red bell pepper into small pieces.

- 1/2 cup chopped carrots.

- 2 tablespoons minced fresh tarragon leaves.

- 1 tablespoon fresh lemon juice

- Salt and pepper.

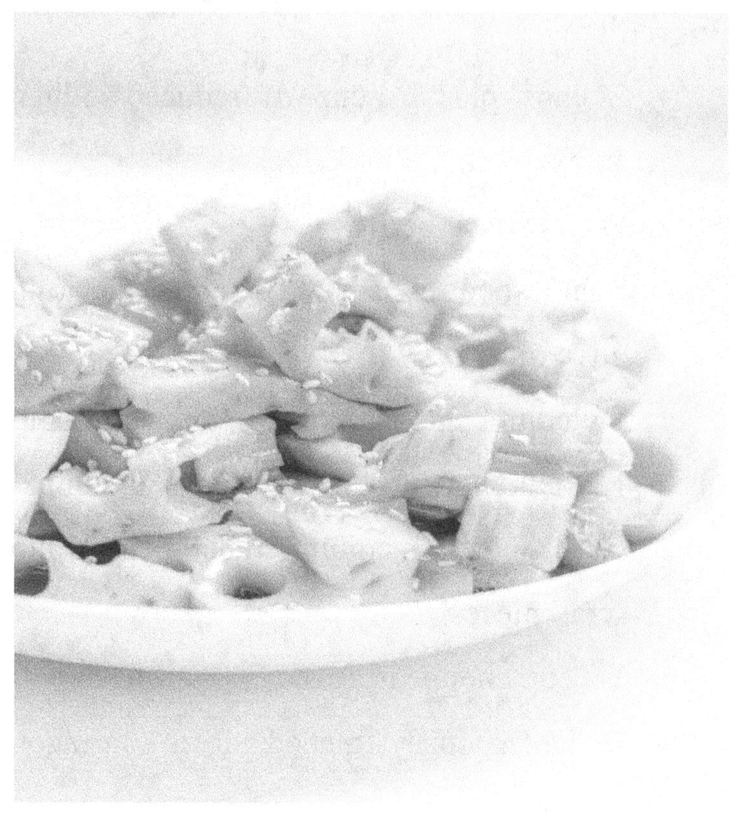

Instructions:

- In a medium saucepan set over high heat, bring 2 cups broth and 2 cups water to a boil. Reduce heat to low and simmer, covered, for 45 to 1 hour. Wheat Berries should be soft but chewy. Drain.

- Meanwhile, heat 1 tablespoon of oil in a medium nonstick skillet over medium heat. Cook the shallot for 3 minutes while stirring.

- Cook for 3 minutes, stirring to coat the asparagus, red pepper, and carrots. Simmer the remaining ½ cup of stock in the skillet.

- In a medium serving bowl, combine drained wheat berries and veggies. Add tarragon, lemon juice, the remaining 1 teaspoon oil, and salt and pepper to taste. Toss to coat. Serve warm or room temperature.

Make Ahead: You may make the salad up to one day in advance. Refrigerate, securely covered.

Serves two.

Nutritional Information:
- 1 serving is 280 calories.
- Vitamin C: one serving.
- Green/yellow vegetables: one serving
- Other vegetables: 1/2 serving.
- Whole grains: one serving.
- Fat: 1/2 serving

Fig and Arugula Salad with Parmesan Shavings

Fresh figs make this an extremely seductive salad; serve it, and romance will be on the menu.

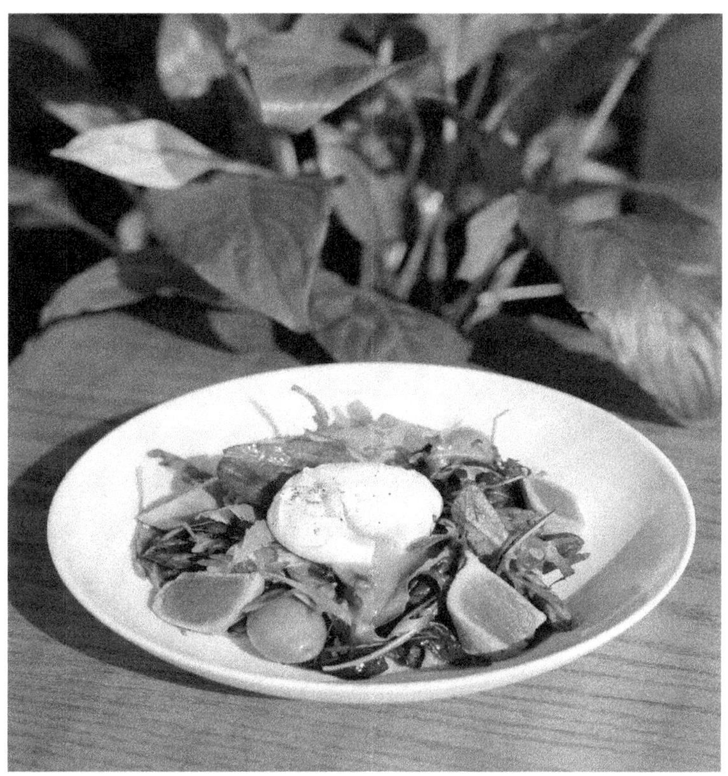

Ingredients:

- One big shallot, minced

- 2 teaspoons of balsamic vinegar.

- 1–2 tablespoons extra-virgin olive oil

- 1 teaspoon of whole grain mustard.

- Salt

- 8 fresh figs sliced in half.

- 4 cups (packed). Arugula, cleaned and thick stems removed.

- Black pepper

- ½ cup Parmesan cheese shavings (about. 2 oz)

Direction:

- In a large salad bowl, combine the shallot, balsamic vinegar, olive oil, mustard, and a touch of salt. Whisk together.

- Add the figs, stir to coat evenly, and set aside for 20 minutes, covered with plastic wrap.

- Toss the figs and arugula together. Season to taste with salt and pepper, and mix thoroughly. Divide the fig salad across two smaller salad dishes, then sprinkle with Parmesan shavings.

Serves two.

Nutritional information: One serving provides:
- Calcium: One serving.
- Vitamin C: 1/2 serving.
- Green leafy and yellow veggies and fruits: two servings.

- Fat content: ½ serve with 1 tablespoon oil, 1 serving with 2.

Steak Salad

There's no need to visit your neighborhood steakhouse. Here's steak and salad on the same platter. Instead of sliced raw mushrooms, use grilled or roasted Portobello mushrooms.

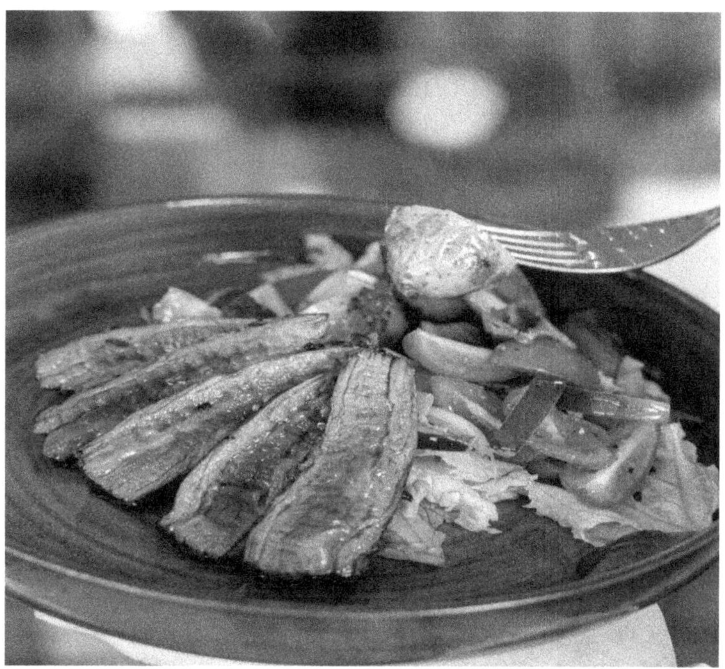

Ingredients:

- Salt and cracked black pepper.

- 1 strip steak or sirloin steak (approximately 1 ¼ inch thick and 12 ounces), fat-trimmed
- Ingredients: 1 teaspoon finely grated lemon zest, 2 tablespoons fresh lemon juice.
- 1-2 tablespoons mayonnaise
- Black pepper
- One medium-sized red onion, cut into ¼-inch thick slices.
- 4 cups (packed) arugula or equivalent fragile greens, with thick stems removed.
- 1 cup, thinly sliced button mushrooms
- 1 roasted red bell pepper (leftover or from a jar), thinly sliced
- ½ cup Parmesan cheese shavings (about. 2 oz)

Direction:

- Preheat the broiler or grill on high.

- Season the steak evenly with salt and cracked pepper.

- Broil or grill the steak for 3 to 5 minutes per side, or until an instant-read meat thermometer registers 160 degrees Fahrenheit.

- Meanwhile, combine the lemon zest, lemon juice, and mayonnaise in a small bowl and whisk together.

- Season with salt and pepper to taste. (If it's too tart for your liking, add another tablespoon of mayonnaise.) Set the dressing aside.

- Transfer the steak to a cutting board, leaving the broiler or grill on. Allow the steak to rest for 5 minutes before slicing into ¼ inch slices. Save the meat juices.

- Broil or grill the onion for 3 minutes per side, or until it is cooked through and slightly browned. Place the sautéed onions, arugula, mushrooms, and bell pepper in a salad dish and swirl to combine.

- Pour the dressing and beef juice over them. Sprinkle Parmesan cheese over the salads and serve.

Serves two.

Nutritional information: One serving provides:

- Protein: 1 ½ serving.

- Calcium: One serving.

- Vitamin C: 2 ½ servings.

- Green leafy and yellow veggies and fruits: three servings.

- Other fruits and vegetables: two portions.

- Fat content: ½ serving with 1 tablespoon mayonnaise, 1 serving with 2 tablespoons.

Shrimp Caesar Salad

Maybe you think of grilled chicken as the typical topper for a Caesar salad, but you'll hail Caesar when this twist on the classic includes a beloved sea creature.

Ingredients:

- Shelled and deveined 12 large shrimp. Use olive oil frying spray.

- Black pepper

- 4 cups shredded romaine lettuce.

- One medium-sized red bell pepper, finely sliced

- 1 cup tiny cherry or grape tomatoes.

- 2 tablespoons Caesar dressing (recipe below)

- 1/2 cup grated Parmesan cheese, or more to taste.

- Two lemon slices for serving.

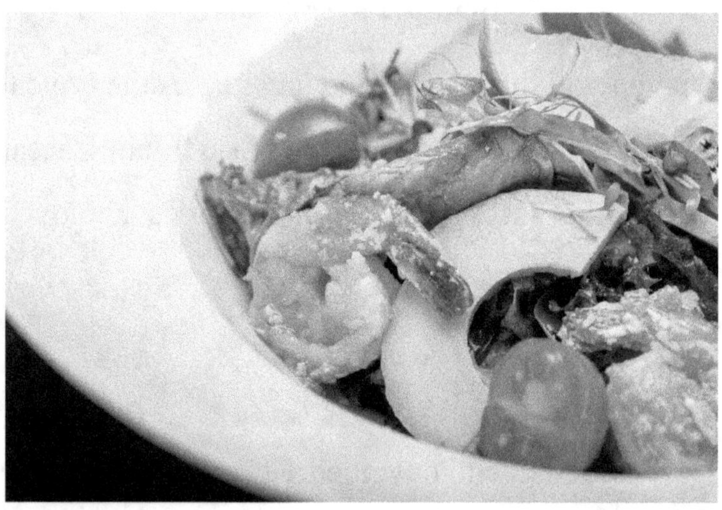

Direction:

- Season the shrimp with black pepper.

- Coat a skillet with olive oil cooking spray and heat it on high. Cook the shrimp until fully cooked, about 4 minutes. Set the shrimp aside.

- In a small bowl, stir together the lettuce, bell pepper, tomatoes, salad dressing, and Parmesan cheese.

- Divide the salad across two salad plates and top with eight shrimp. Serve with lemon wedges and additional Parmesan, if preferred.

Serves two.

Grilled chicken breast is a tried-and-true topping for a Caesar salad. Grilled salmon is another tasty option.

Nutritional Information: One serving (without dressing) provides:

- Protein: One serving.
- Calcium: One serving.
- Vitamin C: four servings.
- Green leafy and yellow veggies and fruits: three servings.

Caesar Dressing

Raw eggs are used to make classic Caesar dressing. This eggless version is ideal for the pregnant gourmet who wants the full flavor of a superb Caesar salad without any problematic additives.

Ingredients:

- 1 tbsp chopped garlic
- 4 teaspoons of fresh lemon juice.
- 2 tbsp of olive oil (or add your desired quantity to taste)
- Two anchovy filets (optional) Drain and coarsely chop. Add 1/4 cup grated Parmesan cheese, or more to taste.
- Salt and cracked black pepper.

Direction:

- In a blender or food processor, combine the garlic, lemon juice, olive oil, anchovies (if using), and Parmesan cheese. Puree until smooth. Season to taste with salt and cracked pepper, and add extra olive oil and/or cheese if preferred.

Makes approximately ½ cup.

Nutritional Information:

- One serving (¼ cup) provides:
- Calcium: 1/2 serving.
- Vitamin C: 1/2 serving.
- Fat: 1 ½ servings.

Fresh tomato slices atop baby greens with grated parmesan and a basic balsamic dressing

A simple salad topped with one of the most adaptable and trustworthy dressings available; triple the recipe and save the remaining dressing for future salads.

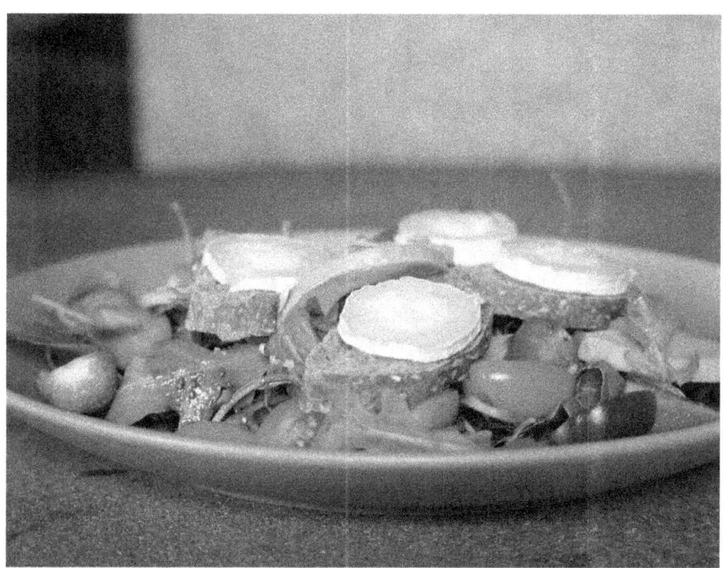

Direction

- For the finest flavor, use extra virgin olive oil in dressings and salads. Regular olive oil works well for cooking.

- In a large salad bowl, combine the shallot, balsamic vinegar, olive oil, mustard, and a touch of salt. Whisk together.

- Add the figs, stir to coat evenly, and set aside for 20 minutes, covered with plastic wrap.

- Toss the figs and arugula together. Season to taste with salt and pepper, and mix thoroughly. Divide the fig salad across two smaller salad dishes, then sprinkle with Parmesan shavings.

Serves two.

Nutritional information: One serving provides:

Calcium: One serving.

Vitamin C: 1/2 serving.

Green leafy and yellow veggies and fruits: two servings.

Fat content: ½ serve with 1 tablespoon oil, 1 serving with 2.

Ingredients:

- Salad: 1 tomato.
- 1 cup lettuce.
- 2 tablespoons of parmesan cheese.

Dressing:

- 2 tablespoons balsamic vinegar.
- 2 teaspoons fresh lemon juice
- One clove garlic, minced

- 1 tablespoon Dijon mustard
- 2 tablespoons extra virgin olive oil.
- Salt and pepper.

Instructions:

In a small resealable container, add the first four dressing ingredients; close and shake to blend. Combine the oil, salt, and pepper; seal the container and shake well. Refrigerate, securely covered. Toss with lettuce and tomato.

Make ahead: Dressing can be made up to five days in advance. Refrigerate, securely covered.

Nutritional Information:

- Salad with 1 tablespoon dressing is 125 calories.
- Vitamin C: one serving.

- Calcium: 1/2 serving.

- Green or yellow vegetables: 1 ½ servings.

- Fat: 1/2 serving

Spinach Strawberry Salad

Here's a quick and easy summer treat. If the onion offends your stomach (or if you plan on kissing after dinner), leave it out; the salad will still be delicious.

Ingredients:

- 4 cups (packed). Baby spinach

- 1 cup sliced fresh strawberries (about. ½ pint).

- 1/2 cup sliced red onion (optional)

- 1/4 cup toasted sliced almonds.

- 2 teaspoons of distilled white vinegar or white wine vinegar.

- 2 tablespoons of canola oil.

- Two tablespoons of white grape juice concentrate, and apple juice concentrate, Splenda, honey, or brown sugar (to taste).

- ½ teaspoon paprika.

- Salt and black pepper.

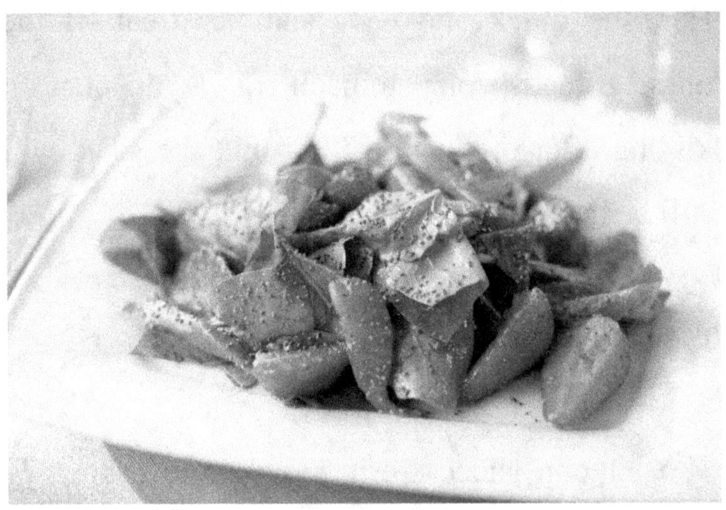

Direction:

- Place the spinach, strawberries, onion (if using), and almonds in a salad bowl.

- In a small bowl, combine the vinegar, oil, grape juice concentrate, and paprika.

- Whisk well. Season with salt and pepper to taste. Toss the salad with enough dressing to cover evenly. Divide the salad into two smaller salad bowls and serve.

Serves two.

Nutritional information: One serving provides:

- Vitamin C: three servings.
- Green leafy and yellow veggies and fruits: two servings.
- Fat: 1 serving.

Shrimp and Mango Salad with Sesame Ginger

Vinaigrette is a simple recipe that requires cleaned and cooked shrimp. It's as delicious with cubes of cooked chicken or turkey.

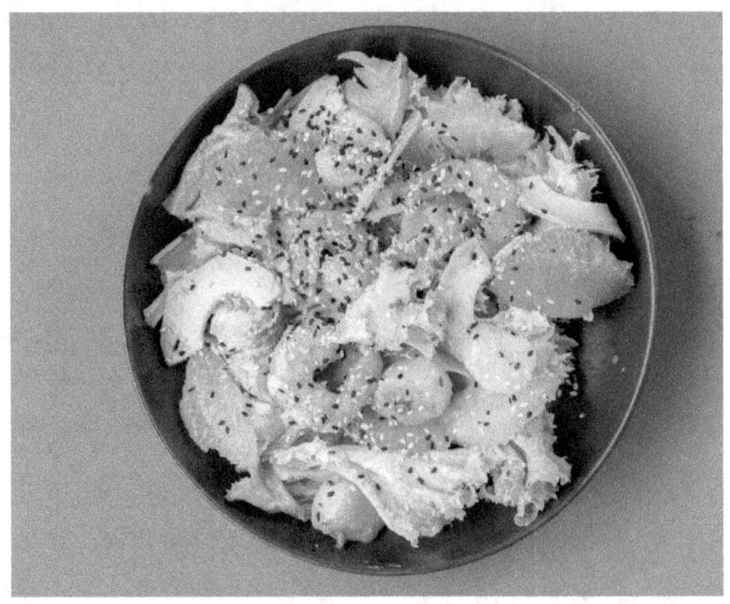

Ingredients:

- 12 big shrimp shelled and deveined.
- 4 cups of packed mesclun or other tender greens.

- Peel and thinly slice one Kirby (pickling) cucumber.
- Sesame Ginger Vinaigrette (recipe below)
- One ripe mango, thinly sliced
- One medium-sized red bell pepper, finely sliced

Direction:

- Steam the shrimp for about 5 minutes, or until they are fully cooked and opaque.

- Put the mesclun and cucumber in a salad bowl.
- Toss in ¼ cup of the Sesame Ginger Vinaigrette. Divide the greens between two salad dishes.

- Place the shrimp, mango, and bell pepper in a salad dish. Toss in enough of the leftover Sesame Ginger Vinaigrette to coat evenly. Carefully top the greens with the already shrimp mixture.

Serves two.

Open, sesame: Toss a couple of tablespoons of sesame seeds (ideally toasted) among the greens for a nutty crunch.

Nutritional information: One serving provides:
- Protein: One serving.
- Vitamin C: two servings.
- Green leafy and yellow veggies and fruits: three servings.
- Other fruits and veggies. ½ serving

Nutty Bulgur Salad

Refrigerate the salad for a few hours before serving to allow the flavors to combine. Shallots provide the mildest onion flavor, but you can use an equivalent quantity of red or Vidalia onion if you want.

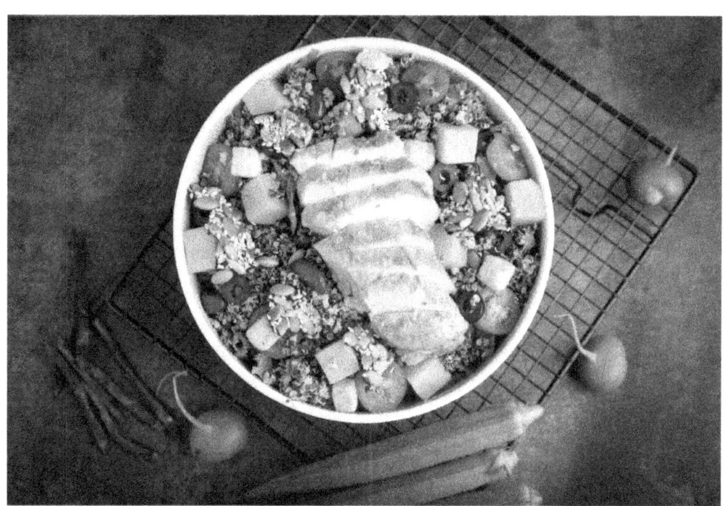

Ingredients:

- 1 cup bulgur wheat.
- 2 teaspoons olive oil.
- One big shallot, minced

- 1 teaspoon cinnamon.

- ½ teaspoon ground cumin

- ½ teaspoon allspice.

- 1/2 cup dried apricots.

- 1/2 cup golden raisins.

- 3 tablespoons minced fresh mint

- 3 tablespoons pine nuts, 1/4 cup orange juice.

- Salt and black pepper.

Instructions:

- Heat 1 1/4 cups of water in a medium saucepan until boiling. Stir in the bulgur. Bring back to a boil, then remove from heat and cover the saucepan.

- Allow to stand for 30 minutes.

- Meanwhile, heating the oil in a small nonstick skillet over medium-low heat. Stir in the shallots and simmer for 3 minutes. Stir in the cinnamon, cumin, and allspice and toast for 1 minute.

- Place the bulgur in a large ceramic bowl. Fold in the shallot combination, apricots, raisins, mint, pine nuts, and orange juice.

- Add salt and pepper to taste.

- Refrigerate until well cooled. Serve cool.

Makes approximately 4 cups.

Make ahead: Make the salad up to three days in advance. Refrigerate, securely covered.

Nutritional Information:

- 1 cup equals 310 calories.
- Protein: less than one serving.
- Other fruits and vegetables: 1/2 serving.
- Consume 1½ servings of whole grains.

Salad with toasted barley, roasted red peppers, and corn with feta cheese

This salad is packed with summer flavors, including red peppers, corn, tomatoes, and basil. Fortunately, this recipe tastes nearly as excellent in the winter, when cooked with frozen corn and cherry tomatoes. Dry-toasting the barley gives it a nutty flavor, but omit this step if you're short on time. You can also avoid roasting the pepper, but the salad will not have the same smokey flavor.

Don't try to replace dried basil; it simply doesn't have the same flavor.

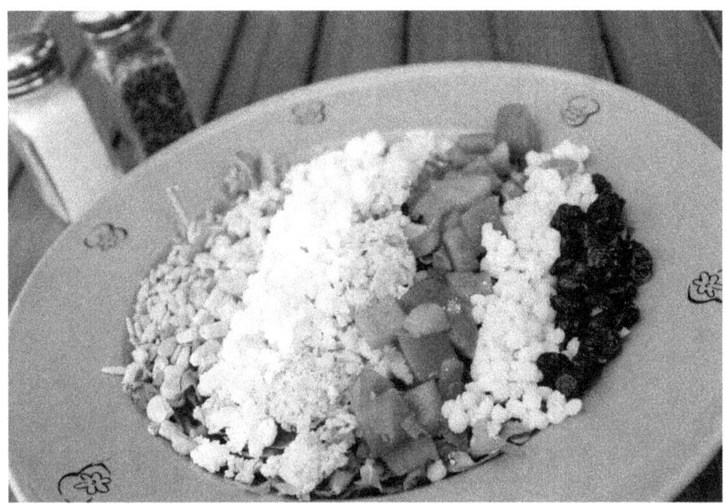

Ingredients

- 1/2 cup pearl barley.

- 1½ cups reduced-sodium chicken broth and 1 medium red bell pepper.

- 2 Tbsp and 1 tsp fresh lime juice

- 1 tablespoon of olive oil.

- Two large plum tomatoes, seeded and sliced.

- 1 cup fresh corn kernels, no need to cook
- 1/4 cup sliced scallions (white and light green sections)
- ¼ cup freshly minced basil leaves
- 2 tablespoons pasteurized feta cheese.

Instructions:

- Toast barley in a big heavy pot over medium heat for 8 minutes, shaking often.

- Bring broth to a boil in the pan. Reduce the heat to low, cover, and simmer for 35 minutes, or until the liquid is absorbed and the barley is soft. Let it cool.

- Meanwhile, grill or broil the bell pepper until it is browned on all sides. Allow to stand for 10 minutes, sealed in a paper bag or covered bowl. Peel, seed, and dice.

- Carefully combine the lime, juice and oil in a small bowl.

- In a large bowl, combine the tomatoes, corn, and scallions. Fold in the bell pepper and cooled barley.

- Add the oil mixture and stir to combine. Season with salt and pepper to taste. Top with feta cheese. Serve at room temperature and garnish with basil.

Serves four.

This Salad can be prepared up to one day in advance. Refrigerate, securely covered.

Nutritional Information:

- 1 serving is 250 calories.
- Vitamin C: 1½ serving
- Green/yellow vegetable: 1/2 serving.
- Other vegetables: 1/2 serving.
- Whole grains: two servings.
- Calcium, lipids, fiber: some

Peppers and Carrots with Homemade Ranch Dressing

It's simple to dress raw veggies with this chilled, creamy dressing prepared with natural ingredients. A quick and easy way to get in some of your daily dozen!

Ingredients:

- ½ cup buttermilk and ¼ cup mayonnaise

- 1/4 cup low-fat yogurt

- 1 clove garlic, minced

- 1 teaspoon fresh lemon juice

- 1 teaspoon of cider vinegar

- 2 tablespoons chopped fresh Italian parsley leaves.

- 2 thinly sliced scallions (both white and light green)

- 1 medium carrot and 1 red or green pepper.

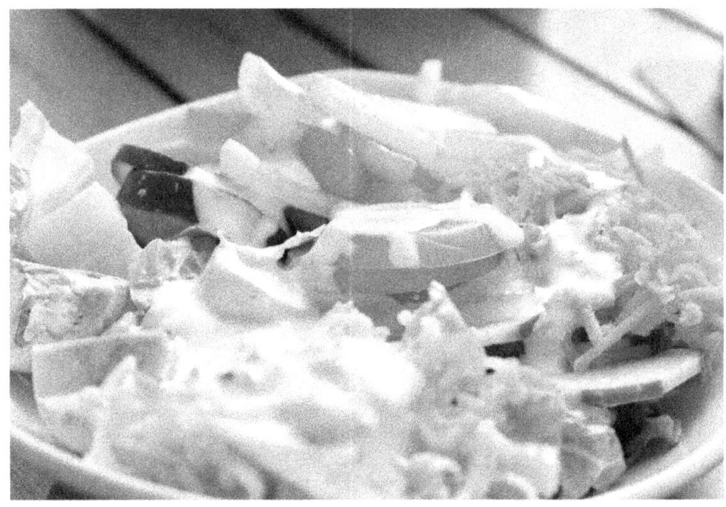

Instructions:

- In a medium bowl, combine all ingredients except the carrot and pepper. Refrigerate tightly covered until ready to serve.

- Cut the carrots and peppers into sticks. Serve with ¼ cup dressing on the side for dipping.

Makes approximately ½ cup dressing.

Make ahead: The dressing can be made up to five days in advance. Refrigerate, securely covered.

Nutritional Information:

- ¼ cup dressing and 1 cup vegetables equal 100 calories.

- Vitamin C: one serving.

- Green/yellow vegetables: two servings

- Calcium, fiber, and fat: some

CHAPTER 5: Nourishing Dinners for Two

These healthy pregnancy meals are ideal for your major meal of the day, when you have more time to plan, make, and consume. As previously noted, it is critical to eat healthy throughout pregnancy to ensure that you and your baby receive all of the necessary energy and minerals. This entails attempting to eat a variety of meals from each of the food groups every day. We have additional advice on how to eat well during pregnancy.

These dish ideas are ideal for your daily dinner. You can make extra portions and store them in the freezer for when you don't have time or want to cook. Always exercise caution when preparing defrosted food.

Meatballs in tomato sauce

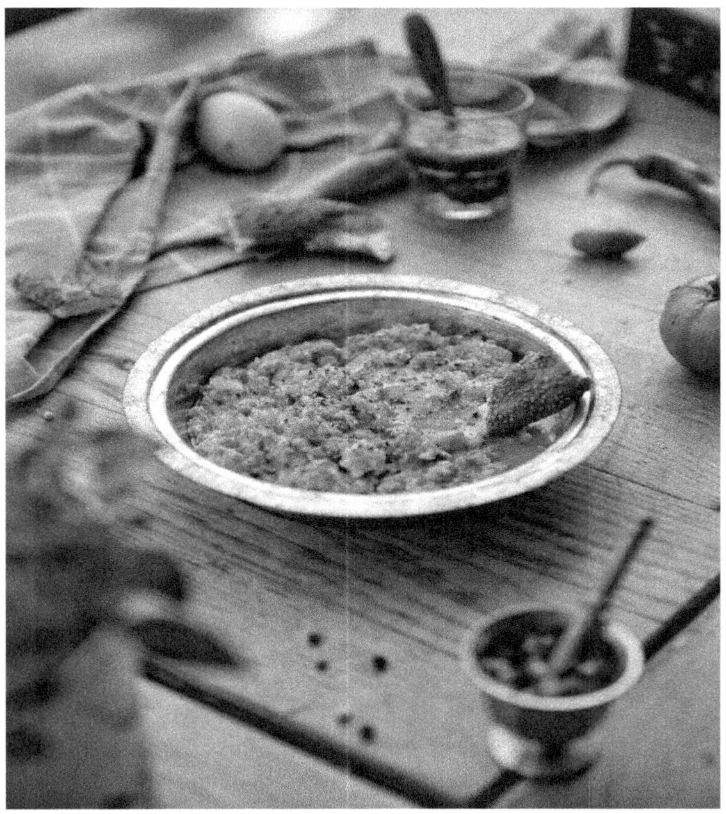

This recipe yields 4 pieces of around 180g.

Ingredients

- 300 g beef mince.
- One egg, beaten

- 1/2 teaspoon of black pepper powder.

- 1/2 tablespoon of vegetable oil.

- One medium onion, finely chopped

- 1 large (400g) can of chopped tomatoes.

Method:

- Use 100ml of water.

- Place the mince, egg, and pepper in a large mixing bowl and well combine with your hands.

- Roll the mixture between your palms to form approximately 12 tiny balls.

- Heat the oil in a frying pan and brown the onions and meatballs.

- Add the tomatoes and water, and cook for 30 minutes.

- Serve alongside mashed potatoes and a couple pieces of broccoli.

African Beef Stew

This recipe yields 4 pieces of around 160g.

Ingredients

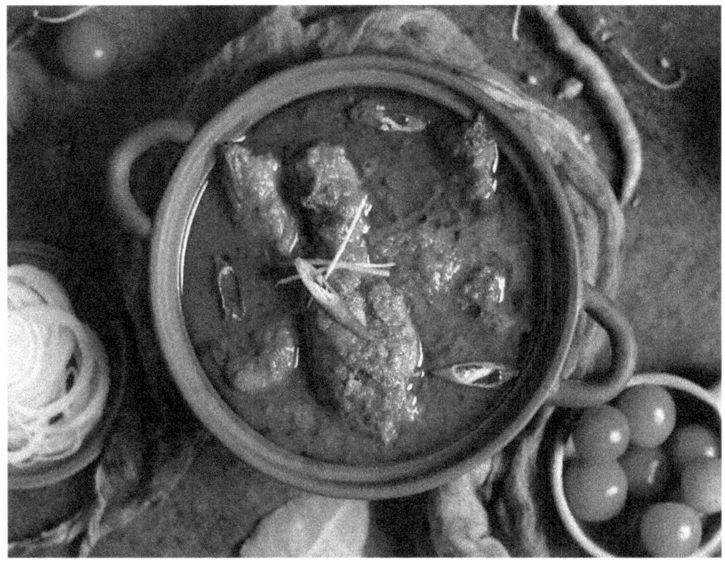

- 350g of lean beef stewing steak.

- 1 tablespoon of vegetable oil.

- 1/2 medium onion coarsely chopped.

- 1/2 teaspoon of fresh root ginger, make it peeled and grated.

- 1 garlic clove, smashed

- 1 small (200g) can of chopped tomatoes.

- 1/2 medium green pepper, coarsely chopped

- 1/2 teaspoon of ground cayenne pepper.

Method:

- 100g chopped spinach leaves.

- Cut the meat into thin pieces.

- Heat the oil over medium heat, then cook the onion without browning.

- Fry the beef, ginger, and garlic until the meat browned.

- Cook for about 40 minutes, stirring in the tomatoes, green pepper, and cayenne pepper until the meat is cooked.

- Cook for a further 5 minutes after adding the spinach.

Serve with a dish of roasted plantains or potatoes.

Tuna and tomato pasta

This recipe yields 4 pieces of around 300g.

Ingredients

- 2 tablespoons of vegetable oil.

- 1 medium, diced onion

- 1 clove garlic, coarsely chopped

- 1 1/2 large (400g) cans chopped tomatoes with seasonings (total weight 600g)

- 1 teaspoon of sugar.

- 250g dried pasta in shapes like penne

- Drain 1 1/2 cans (185g) of tuna in spring water (210g drained weight). (Whenever feasible, buy seafood from sustainable sources.)

Method:

- Gradually heat the oil and sauté the onions in a saucepan until it's tender.

- Cook for a further minute after adding the chopped garlic.

- Bring the diced tomatoes and sugar to a boil.

- Reduce the heat and let it simmer without a lid for about 12 minutes.

- Use the package direction in the pasta to cook it in boiling water.

- Flake the drained tuna with a fork and put it into the pasta sauce to heat thoroughly.

- Drain the cooked pasta thoroughly and return it to the saucepan. Gently Pour the sauce over the pasta and carefully stir till properly mixed.

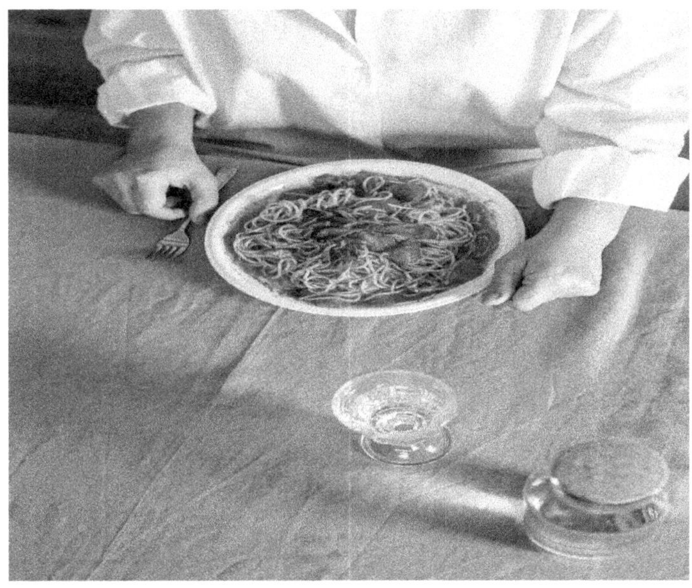

Serve with a side salad of lettuce, tomatoes, and cucumber to complete your 5-a-day.

Limit your tuna consumption as it contains higher levels of mercury compared to other seafood. If you consume too much mercury, it can harm your unborn child. You should consume no more than two tuna steaks (about 140g cooked or 170g raw) or four medium-size cans of tuna (approximately 140g drained) every week.

Homemade fish fingers

This recipe yields 4 pieces of around 90g.

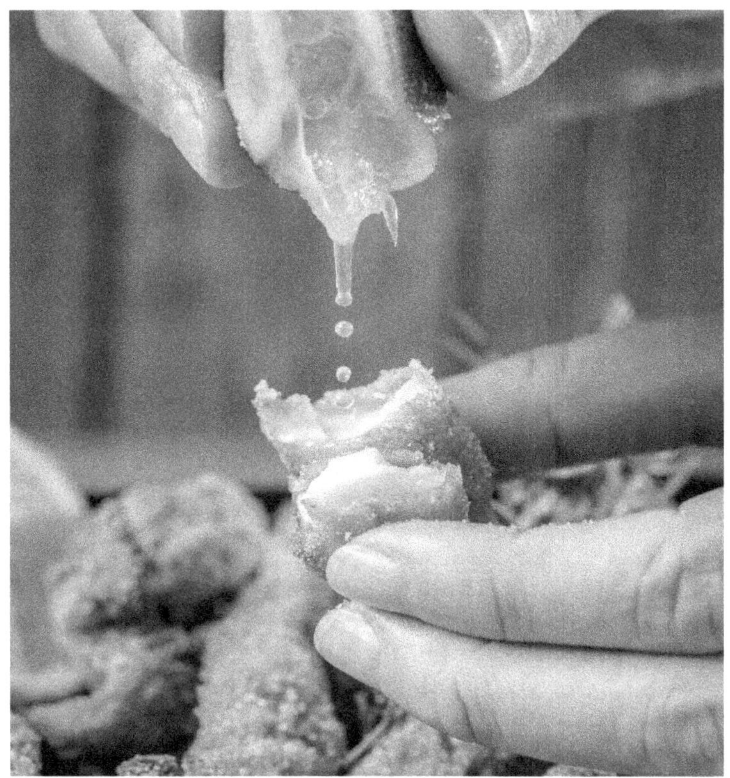

Ingredients:

- 350g salmon or cod filet (fresh or frozen, properly defrosted) (Whenever feasible, buy seafood from sustainable sources.)

- 2 eggs

- 3 pieces of bread, crumbed

- A side salad with lettuce, tomatoes, and cucumber.

Method:

- Preheat the oven to 190°C / 375°F/Gas 5.

- Cut the salmon fillet into 12 evenly spaced strips.

- To prepare an egg wash, beat the eggs together in a small bowl.

- Dip the salmon strips in egg wash, then wrap them in breadcrumbs until completely coated.

- Place the coated strips on a baking pan and bake for 15 minutes.

- A side salad with lettuce, tomatoes, and cucumber.

When serving fish, make sure to remove any bones.

Jerk chicken with rice, peas, and callaloo

This recipe yields 4 pieces of around 100g.

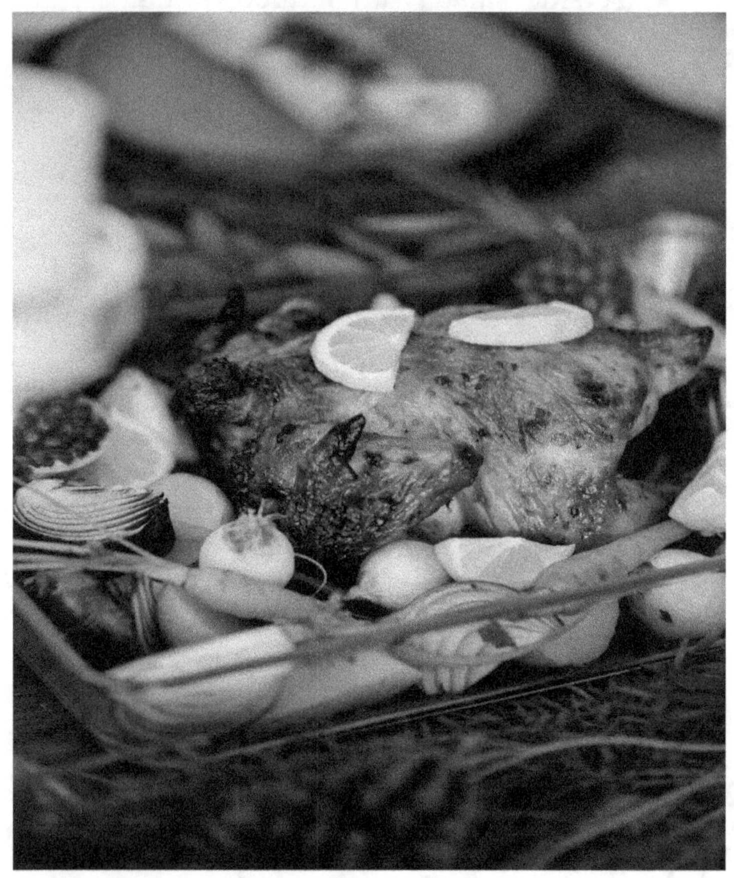

Ingredients:

- 4 chicken breasts with skin removed.

- For jerk seasoning:

- 1 tablespoon of ground allspice.

- 1 tablespoon of dried thyme.

- 2 teaspoons of cayenne pepper.

- 2 tablespoons garlic granules

- 1 teaspoon of ground black pepper.

- 1 teaspoon ground cinnamon.

- 3 tablespoons of vegetable oil.

Method:

- Put the chicken in a shallow basin.

- Combine the jerk seasoning ingredients and then pour them over the chicken breasts.

- Stir them around to coat them with the mixture. Then cover it and marinate in the refrigerator for a minimum of an hour.

- Remove the chicken from the refrigerator and cook for 2 minutes on each side under a hot grill. Reduce the heat and grill for a further 20 to 25 minutes, flipping occasionally.

Serve with rice, peas, and some callaloo.

Rice with Peas

This recipe yields 4 pieces of around 180g.

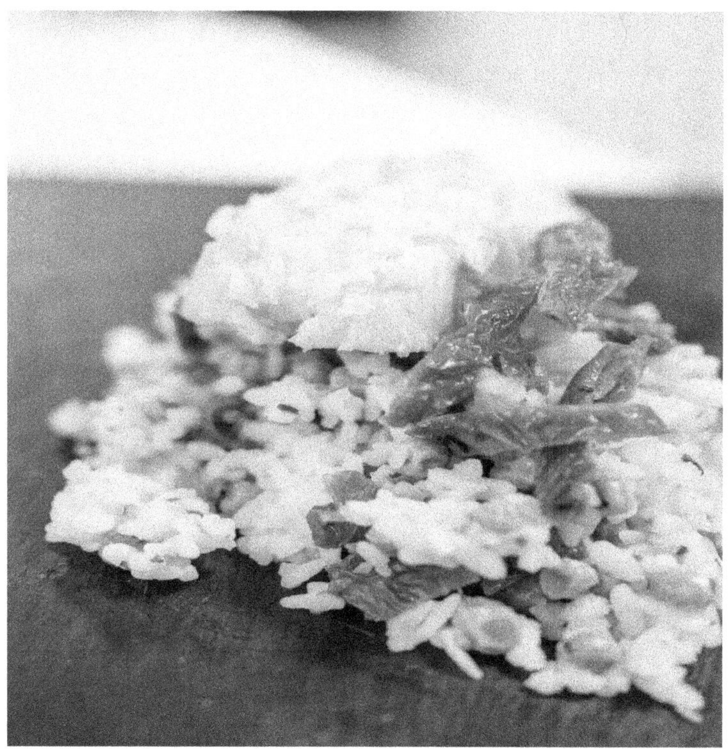

Ingredients:

- 1 small can (220g) washed and drained kidney beans.
- 1 teaspoon dried thyme.

- 1 teaspoon of white pepper.

- Dice 1/2 small onion and mix with 400ml of water.

- 200 gram long grain rice

Method:

- In a saucepan, combine all of the ingredients except the rice and heat until boiling.

- Add the rice and stir.

- Boil quickly for 3 to 4 minutes, then reduce heat and simmer gently for 10 to 12 minutes, stirring periodically, until the rice is cooked.

Vegetable curry, lentil dahl, and rice

This recipe yields 4 pieces of around 200g.

Vegetable Curry Ingredients:

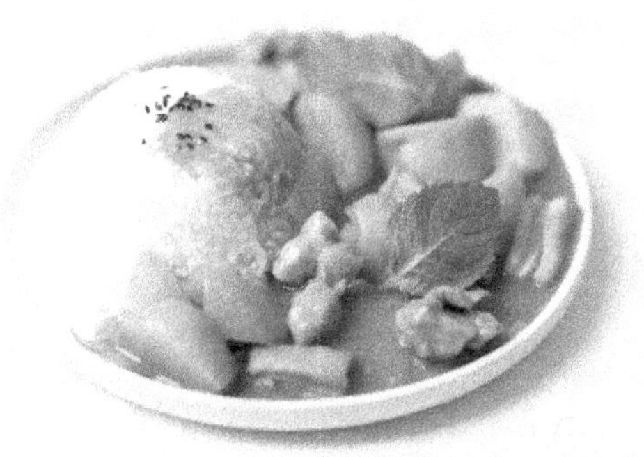

- 1 tablespoon of vegetable oil.

- One medium onion, peeled and sliced

- 2 tbsp curry powder

- 1 clove garlic, coarsely chopped, 150ml water

- Two medium carrots, peeled and sliced

- 1/2 small head of cauliflower (florets only)
- One big potato, peeled and cubed
- 1 small (200g) can of sweetcorn (approx. 160g when drained).
- 1/2 small (150g) carton of low-fat natural yogurt

Method:

- In a saucepan, heat the oil and sauté the onion until it softens and browns.

- Cook for 1 minute with the curry powder and garlic.

- Add water.

- Bring the carrots, cauliflower, potatoes, and sweet corn to a boil.

- Reduce heat, cover it, and let it simmer for at least 15 minutes.

- Remove from heat and mix in the yoghurt. Return the pan to low heat and cook for 2 minutes.

Lentil Dal

This recipe yields 4 pieces of around 80g.

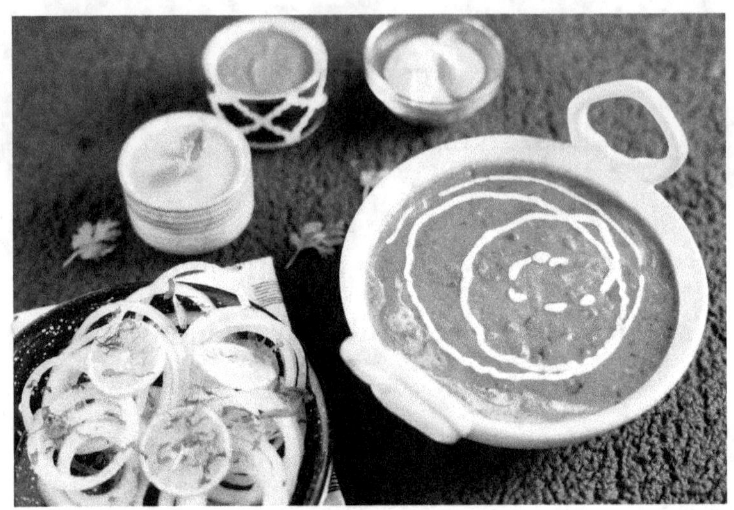

Ingredients:

- 150 g split red lentils, 1 tablespoon vegetable oil.
- 1 teaspoon of cumin seeds.
- 1/2 small onion, diced.
- 1 clove garlic, coarsely chopped
- Ingredients: 1/2 teaspoon ground ginger, 1 teaspoon mild chili powder.

- 1 teaspoon ground turmeric.

- 1 small, chopped tomato

- 150 ml water

Method:

- Boil the lentils in water until tender. Drain any excess water.

- Heat the vegetable oil in a big pan and cook the cumin seeds for about a minute, or until they 'pop'.

- Fry the onion, garlic, ginger, chilli powder, and turmeric for a few minutes, until the onions soften.

- Cook the cooked lentils, diced tomato, and water in the pan for 5 to 10 minutes, stirring occasionally.

Jacket potato with roasted veggie and tomato filling, including vegetable sticks

This recipe yields 4 pieces of around 130g.

Ingredients:

- 1 medium courgette, 8 medium mushrooms.
- 1 medium onion and 1 small red pepper.
- One little yellow pepper.
- 1 teaspoon of dry mixed herbs.
- 1 tablespoon of vegetable oil.
- 1 can (400g) Chopped tomatoes (optional). 60g of grated Cheddar or vegan cheese

Method:

- Preheat the oven to 180C / 350F / Gas 4.
- Cut the veggies into pieces.

- Place all of the vegetables, except the tomatoes, on a baking dish, sprinkle with the mixed herbs, and drizzle with the oil.

- Roast for 25 minutes, until soft. Add the tomato, combine well, and simmer for another 5 minutes.

- Sprinkle it with cheese, or vegan cheese, right before serving.

CHAPTER 6: Snacks and Treats to Satisfy Cravings

Whether you call them snacks or micro meals, eating tiny nibbles throughout the day can be a healthy and convenient way to receive your daily intake of key nutrients, particularly during pregnancy.

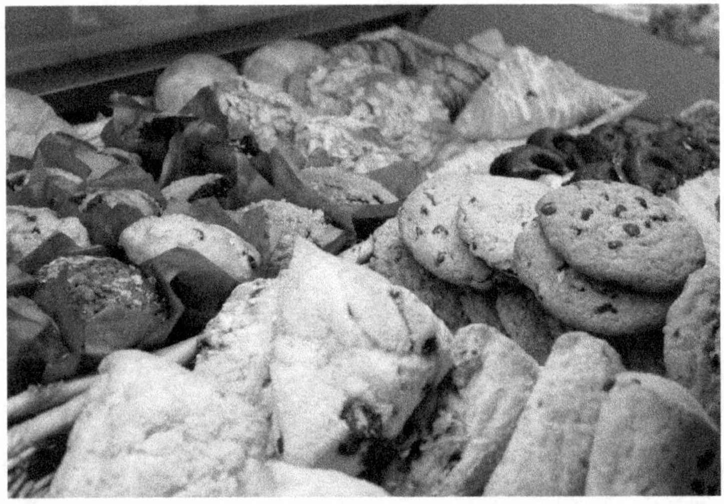

When you're dealing with stomach concerns like nausea and food aversions in the early stages of pregnancy, little bites are easier to swallow. Healthy snacks are also a fantastic method to gain sustenance later in pregnancy, when you feel stuffed and unable to eat another meal after just a few forkfuls.

Snacks, too, are an effective kind of nutritional insurance. While your calorie requirements increase during pregnancy (500 more per day by the third trimester), it is more important than ever to use those extra calories to provide your body with key nutrients that aid in your baby's development, particularly protein, folate, calcium, vitamin D, DHA (omega-3 fatty acid), iodine, and iron.

So, what should you eat these days to keep your energy levels up between meals while also providing your child with extra nutrition? Good pregnancy snacks are tasty, healthful, and full, and there are many options. Here are some of the greatest snack ideas for pregnancy, regardless of the flavors you crave.

Healthy dry snacks during pregnancy

Yes, a cup of yogurt or a smoothie can be a good pick-me-up. But occasionally you need a dry option that is portable and can sit in your backpack for hours without being chilled. In addition to being convenient, dry snacks frequently contain entire grains, nuts, and dried fruit, making them an excellent way to increase fiber in your diet and prevent pregnancy constipation, as well as load up on protein and B vitamins. Dry foods are also quite easy to consume while you're feeling sick.

Trail mix: The nut, seed, and dried fruit combination contains protein, healthy fats, and fiber to keep you going for hours. Add additional exciting ingredients like cashews, pumpkin seeds, dried cherries, or dark chocolate chips.

Granola bars: Think of them as trail mix bars with the addition of robust, fiber-rich oats. Some granola bars can be as sweet as desserts, so choose alternatives prepared with genuine fruits and nuts.

Whole-grain pretzels: Check the label to be sure yours are prepared with whole grains. If the first ingredient listed includes the word "whole" (such as "whole wheat" or "whole oats"), you're generally okay to go.

Fresh fruit and nut butter package: Bananas and apples can be stored at room temperature. A spoonful of nut butter on top provides protein and healthy fats, keeping you satisfied for **longer:** Look for single-serving nut butter packages that you can drop in your bag and go.

Air-popped corn: popcorn is a high-fiber whole grain. Look for air-popped choices and customize with your own seasonings, such as cinnamon or savory nutritional yeast.

Healthy protein snacks during pregnancy

Protein is essential for your baby's growth and development, but it will also help keep your blood sugar levels consistent, allowing you to stay fueled longer and avoid low blood sugar symptoms such as headaches, nausea, and irritability.

Hummus with whole wheat crackers: The chickpea dip contains protein and healthy lipids, while the crackers provide healthful carbohydrates. For a larger appetite, include some sliced raw vegetables and a handful of olives.

Edamame: The tasty soybean pods are high in protein, fiber, iron, folate, and magnesium. To enhance the flavor, microwave the pods and season with salt and sesame seeds.

One handful of nuts: Nuts may be nature's perfect snack due to their high protein, fiber, and healthy fat content. Each type of nut has its own nutritional benefits (almonds include calcium, walnuts have omega-3s, and peanuts contain vitamin E), so eat a variety.

Roasted chickpeas: They're crispy and flavorful like chips, but much more nutritious, with plenty of protein, fiber, and iron. Make your own by baking canned, drained, and rinsed chickpeas with olive oil and your chosen seasonings until crispy, or purchase them ready-made. Are you feeling extra hungry? Prepare a snack dish with roasted chickpeas, cherry tomatoes, and a few cubes of feta cheese.

Hard boiled eggs: Cook a large batch on the weekend, and you'll have a ready-made snack all week. Eggs are high in protein and contain vitamin D, which helps your baby's bones and teeth develop.

Healthy calcium-rich pregnancy snacks

Getting 1,000 milligrams every day is essential for good bones and teeth, both for your kid and yourself. Meeting your nutritional needs at mealtime is not always simple, but calcium-rich snacks can help fill the gap.

More Healthy Eating Tips:

Plain yogurt and fruit: Yogurt contains protein, calcium, and probiotics, which may prevent pregnancy-related constipation. Choosing plain over flavored alternatives will save you a lot of extra sugar; instead, add a healthy amount of sweetness with fresh fruit like berries, chopped mango, or diced apple.

String Cheese: These pre-wrapped bits are ideal for grabbing and eating on the move, and each stick contains around 200 milligrams of calcium. For a more satisfying option, try string cheese with whole grain crackers or wrapped in a whole wheat tortilla.

Cottage cheese: A cup contains approximately 250 milligrams of calcium and a whopping 24 grams of protein. Like yogurt, it's best to stick with simple types and add more flavor yourself. Mix in chopped fruit, sprinkle with honey or cinnamon, or season with salt and lemon juice and serve as a dip for vegetables.

Whole grain cereal with milk: A cup of low-fat milk has 300 milligrams of calcium and 8 grams of protein, and when combined with whole grain cereal, the bone-building beverage becomes a substantial snack or mini-meal. Choose cereals with less than 10 grams of added sugar and at least 3 grams of fiber per serving.

Fruit smoothie with milk: Simple combinations such as banana, almond butter, and milk are easy to drink when you're feeling sick. If you want to add more taste, try frozen cherries with cocoa powder, mango and pineapple, or berries with peanut butter.

Healthy, delicious pregnancy snacks

It is quite acceptable to indulge yourself to the occasional cookie or brownie. However, if your sweet tooth appears on a frequent basis, it's a good idea to keep a few healthier (but still enjoyable) options handy.

Medjool dates and almond butter: Dates are truly nature's candy, being both sweet and sticky. Dunk the dates in protein-packed almond butter for an extra layer of sweetness and fullness.

Frozen banana "ice cream" with chopped almonds: In a food processor, blend a chopped, frozen banana until smooth to create a creamy, naturally sweet ice cream that tastes exactly like the genuine thing. Add chopped walnuts and a cherry for a sundae-like dessert.

Whole grain toast with nut butter and chocolate chips: Spread a spoonful of peanut or almond butter on a slice of whole grain toast, then top with a tablespoon of small dark chocolate chips.

Dark chocolate and clementine: Aim for chocolate with 70 to 85 percent cacao. A higher cocoa content indicates that your chocolate will have more nutrients (such as iron and magnesium) and less added sugar. A one-ounce square is an ideal serving size.

Frozen grapes: This frosty delicacy is ideal for those who want a sweet snack but aren't really hungry. Frozen grapes are pleasant and vitamin-rich, but because they contain neither protein or fat, they are not particularly full on their own.

Healthy nighttime snacks during pregnant

Do you suffer from a rumbling stomach before going to bed? Choose a light, easy-to-digest meal with nutrients that can help you fall asleep.

Whole grain cereal with milk: The combination of complex carbohydrates and protein will make you feel tired. Again, stick with cereals that contain less than 10 grams of sugar per serving. Not only are they more nutritious, but consuming a lot of sugar soon before bed may keep you awake.

Cottage cheese and raspberries: Lean protein sources, such as cottage cheese, contain tryptophan, an amino acid that can cause drowsiness. In addition to its sweetness, raspberries provide a natural source of the sleep-promoting hormone melatonin.

Whole wheat peanut butter toast with banana: The complex carb-protein combination may induce sleep, especially if you include a few slices of banana, another melatonin-rich fruit.

Warm milk with cinnamon: Warm milk is more than just calming; the National Sleep Foundation suggests a correlation between milk's tryptophan and melatonin content and better sleep. Cinnamon provides a delicious sweet accent, but you could also use ground nutmeg or cardamom.

One handful of walnuts: In addition to protein, healthy fats, and omega-3s, walnuts can increase melatonin levels in your blood, allowing you to sleep better.

Snacks to avoid while pregnant

The greatest pregnancy snacks are nutrient-dense selections that keep you energized while giving much-needed vitamins and minerals to you and your growing baby. So it's worth storing up on a variety of healthy foods to keep on hand. While there's nothing wrong with the occasional treat, the foods listed below are rich in calories and low in nutrients, but lack the satiating fiber, protein, and complex carbohydrates that keep you full:

- Cookies, cakes, or sweet baked items
- Candy
- Ice cream
- Potato chips
- Sodas, sweetened teas, and sugary juices
- Sugary coffee beverages.

Of course, you'll want to avoid the standard things that are prohibited during pregnancy, such as raw seafood, undercooked meat, deli meat, undercooked eggs, unpasteurized cheeses or juice, and alcohol.

Healthy snacking suggestions for pregnant ladies

Snacks are essential for remaining satisfied and energized when pregnant, but you probably don't have the time to plan or prepare them. Some techniques to make smart snacking easier:

- Opt for a combination approach. A well-balanced snack with protein, complex carbohydrates, and healthy fats will keep you content for longer, preventing you from craving another bite half an hour later.

- Keep your kitchen supplied. Prepare a range of healthful options, including fresh fruit, almonds, plain yogurt, cheese, whole grain crackers, nut butter, and hummus.

- Prepare grab-and-go snacks ahead of time. Choose two or three snacks for the week, prepare a large batch, then separate them into individual servings to drop in your bag as you leave or grab for when the munchies strike. Prepare a batch of trail mix, boil a dozen eggs, and season a large bowl of popcorn before dividing into single-size baggies.

- Keep your snacking needs in perspective. Remember that you probably won't need any more calories in the first trimester, 300-350 extra calories in the second trimester, and 500 extra calories in the third trimester. Don't bother about tracking calories. Listening to your appetite and storing up on nutritious foods will help you stay on track.

Snacks can be a lifesaver when you're pregnant, both for maintaining energy and slipping extra nutrients into your diet. The goal is to remain with wholesome selections. Here's to wise and healthy snacking!

CHAPTER 7: Celebrating Milestones with Special Occasion Recipes

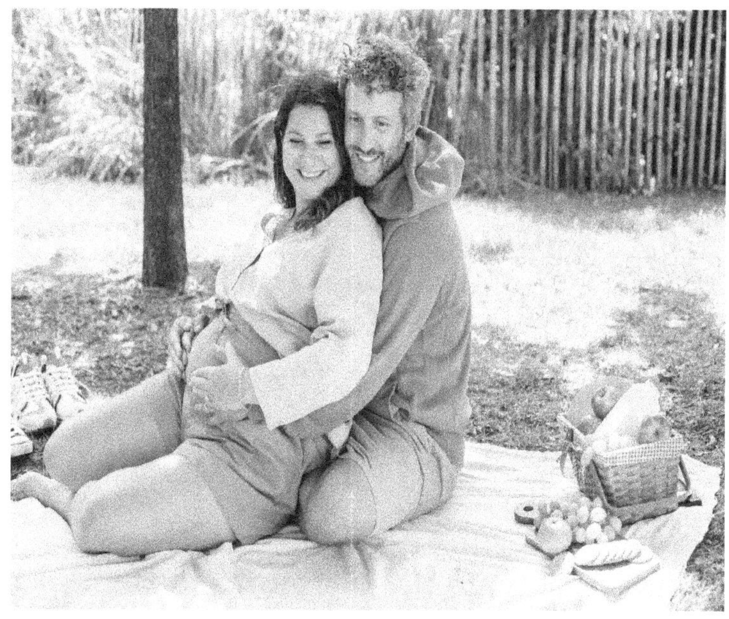

Celebrating pregnancy milestones is a wonderful way to treasure and appreciate the journey of parenthood. Whether it's the first flutter of movement, a crucial milestone in the baby's development, or a simple yet treasured date night, commemorating these events with special occasion dishes adds an extra dimension of joy and meaning to the experience.

Consider preparing a nice lunch to mark those unforgettable achievements. It's more than simply the cuisine; it's about creating an experience that will become a treasured memory in the fabric of your family's history. These special occasion meals are more than just dishes; they express the love and excitement that surrounds your child's approaching arrival.

.

Consider a romantic supper for two, with a thoughtfully prepared cuisine that represents the love and connection between the parents-to-be. Consider a nicely laid table with candlelight, soft music playing in the background, and a food that not only delights the taste senses but also reflects the significance of the occasion. These recipes are created with the concept that certain milestones deserve to be commemorated in a unique way.

Small successes and ordinary delights ought to be celebrated as much as major milestones. Imagine surprising your partner with a delicious breakfast in bed to celebrate a good night's sleep, or making a special snack to commemorate a great pregnancy check-up. These recipes are intended to elevate the ordinary into the extraordinary, bringing a touch of culinary magic to the everyday moments of pregnancy.

Finally, honoring milestones with special occasion meals is about instilling a feeling of occasion and respect for the journey ahead. It's a reminder that every step, no matter how small, is part of the magnificent drama unfolding as you prepare to welcome your child into the world.

CONCLUSION

To summarize, "Pregnancy Cookbook for First Time Dads" is more than simply a cookbook; it's a passionate guide for first-time parents embarking on the magnificent journey of fatherhood. This book will help you grasp the fundamentals of nutrition for mom and baby, stock your pantry with dad-friendly products, and create delicious meals for every occasion.

This cookbook contains more than simple recipes; it is a celebration of love, connection, and the joy of preparing nutritious meals for your growing family. Each dish is prepared with care and intention, transforming the kitchen into a haven of comfort, laughter, and shared memories.

Whether you're making a quick and healthy breakfast, packing energizing lunches for mom-to-be, or indulging in satisfying snacks to satisfy pregnancy cravings, "Pregnancy Cookbook for First Time Dads" provides plenty of inspiration and guidance to help you navigate the culinary aspect of fatherhood with confidence and flair.

So, as you embark on this culinary adventure, keep in mind that every meal prepared with love benefits the health and pleasure of both mother and child. From celebrating milestones with special occasion meals to appreciating the everyday moments of pregnancy, make the kitchen a source of nourishment, connection, and joy as you prepare to welcome your baby into the world. Happy cooking, Dad!

REVIEW PAGE

Dear Reader,

I hope you're well. I'm writing to seek your valuable opinion on my just published book, "Pregnancy Cookbook for First Time Dads". As a reader, your feedback is extremely valuable to me, and I would enjoy hearing your comments on the book.

As you read "Pregnancy Cookbook for First Time Dads," I'd love to hear your thoughts about it. Was the content helpful? Did you find it educational or enjoyable? Which portions of the book did you find most useful? Furthermore, I'd like to hear any suggestions you have for enhancement or areas where you believe the book may be better. Your feedback will not only help me assess how the book is being received, but will also inform future revisions and projects. Your candid feedback is vital in guiding the direction of my work and ensuring that I continue to provide content that resonates with readers like you.

I appreciate you for taking out time to express your opinions. Your advice is very appreciated, and I hope to hear from you soon.

Best Regards,

Eve C. Bird